Anti-Inflammatory Cookbook for Beginners

Boost Immune Health, Reduce Pain and Body Inflammation and Achieve Ideal Weight with **Easy Diet Tips and Delicious Recipes**

28-Day Clean Eating Meal Plan

by Lillian Hudson

Table of Contents

Introduction

Welcome to the "Anti-Inflammatory Cookbook for Beginners"!

This book is designed to help you combat inflammation, which may be may be quietly undermining your well-being and causing issues like fatigue, joint pain, and digestive discomfort. Through practical and easy-to-follow recipes, this cookbook aims to alleviate these problems and enhance your overall wellness. You'll find a collection of accessible, research-backed recipes specifically created to reduce inflammation and boost your health. It will guide you through dietary changes that overtime will lead you to a revitalized, energetic life, significantly improving your happiness and well-being.

We begin our journey with "Understanding Inflammation," a foundational chapter that explains the science behind inflammation. You'll learn how certain foods can either trigger or reduce inflammation, equipping you with the knowledge to make informed dietary choices that promote healing.

Each chapter builds on this understanding, showing how nutrition directly affects your body's inflammatory responses. By following the principles outlined in this book, you can address immediate and chronic health concerns and establish a foundation for disease-free life. You'll discover how to incorporate delicious, anti-inflammatory meals into your daily routine, what to watch out for in common ingredients and an easy meal plan that will transform not only your diet but also your overall health.

Imagine starting each day with renewed energy, feeling invigorated and ready to thrive. This cookbook is designed to make this vision a reality, providing you with the right tools to achieve significant health improvements. Join me on this journey to unlock the power of an anti-inflammatory diet, transform your eating habits and the way you feel, and start living your best life! Welcome to your new beginning!

Chapter 1: Understanding Inflammation

What Exactly is Inflammation?

Inflammation is the body's instinctual response to threats such as injuries and infections, crucial for survival. It mobilizes the immune system, sending white blood cells and chemical messengers to affected areas to promote healing. This is visible when you experience redness or swelling after a cut or a scrape, which is acute inflammation acting as your body's first line of defense to protect itself from harm, whether due to injury, infection, or irritation. It starts when immune cells secrete inflammatory mediators like histamines and prostaglandins, which enhance blood flow to the affected area. This process manifests as the acute inflammation symptoms we all recognize: redness, heat, swelling, and pain.

However, when inflammation persists beyond the initial response to danger, it transforms into chronic inflammation. This prolonged form can stealthily damage your body, often without noticeable symptoms at first. Over time, chronic inflammation can erode tissues and alter cellular processes, contributing to major health issues such as cardiovascular diseases, type 2 diabetes, cancers, and Alzheimer's disease. The insidious nature of chronic inflammation means it can undermine health by perpetually stressing the body's systems, leading to gradual and often irreversible damage.

At this stage, without going too deep, the dual role of inflammation is essential for healing minor injuries and infections but can become a persistent threat when it transitions into a chronic state. Grasping the intricate balance of inflammation and its effects on our bodies is crucial for anyone aiming to optimize their health.

Long-Term Effects on the Body from Inflammation

The darker side of inflammation occurs when it lingers, becoming chronic. This form of inflammation can be triggered by long-term exposure to irritants like pollution, unresolved infections, or as part of an autoimmune condition where the body mistakenly attacks healthy tissues. Chronic inflammation often flies under the radar, lacking the obvious symptoms of its acute counterpart, yet it can wreak havoc on the body by promoting DNA damage and cell death. This contributes significantly to diseases such as rheumatoid arthritis, cardiovascular diseases, and certain cancers.

For example, in the context of nutrition, consuming excessive amounts of processed foods and sugars can continuously provoke the immune system, leading to low-grade chronic inflammation. This type of diet-induced inflammation can accelerate plaque buildup in arteries, a precursor to heart disease.

Common Triggers of Chronic Inflammation

Chronic inflammation acts as a silent saboteur within the body, often triggered by seemingly harmless daily habits and environmental factors. In this section, we will explore the primary factors—ranging from dietary choices to lifestyle habits and environmental exposures—that contribute to the sustained inflammatory responses capable of undermining long-term health.

- ○ **Dietary Choices**: The standard Western diet, rich in processed foods, refined sugars, and unhealthy fats, significantly contributes to the rise in inflammation. These foods not only disrupt gut health but also cause an overproduction of pro-inflammatory cytokines, exacerbating inflammatory responses.

- ○ **Lifestyle Factors**: Sedentary behavior, chronic stress, and insufficient sleep are potent enablers of chronic inflammation. These lifestyle habits disturb the body's natural balance, enhancing inflammatory processes. Regular physical activity, effective stress management, and quality sleep are essential in mitigating these effects.

- ○ **Environmental Influences**: Prolonged exposure to environmental pollutants, such as industrial chemicals and urban smog, can trigger inflammatory responses. These toxins can invade the body's systems, prompting a chronic immune reaction.

- ○ **Persistent Infections and Autoimmune Conditions**: Infections that linger or aren't fully resolved can cause the immune system to remain in a constant state of alert, leading to prolonged inflammation. Additionally, autoimmune diseases, where the immune system mistakenly attacks healthy body tissue, can cause continuous inflammatory responses.

By understanding the underlying causes and mechanisms of chronic inflammation, individuals are empowered to proactively manage their health. Strategic modifications in diet, improvements in lifestyle choices, and mitigation of environmental exposures constitute essential tactics in this endeavor. Prioritizing anti-inflammatory foods, integrating consistent physical activity, effectively managing stress, and circumventing detrimental environmental influences can significantly diminish the risk and severity of chronic inflammation. Such proactive management not only forestalls disease but also fosters a healthier, more dynamic existence. For practical guidance on implementing these strategies, the subsequent chapters on The 28-Day Clean Meal Plan and The Health Journal are designed to equip readers with structured, practical tools that aid in adopting and maintaining an anti-inflammatory lifestyle.

The Connection Between Diet and Inflammation

Without a doubt diet plays a pivotal role in influencing your body's functions and overall well-being, with a profound impact on inflammation. The foods we eat can either provoke or prevent inflammation. Diets high in processed foods, refined carbohydrates (like white bread and pastries), unhealthy fats, and added sugars are major contributors to inflammation. These food components lead to the release of pro-inflammatory molecules such as cytokines—small proteins that aid cell-to-cell communication in immune responses and stimulate the movement of cells towards sites of inflammation. Similarly, eicosanoids—lipid compounds involved in inflammatory responses—can also be elevated by consuming the wrong types of foods, exacerbating conditions like arthritis, asthma, and other inflammatory diseases. In contrast, an anti-inflammatory diet can significantly reduce the ill effects of chronic inflammation. This diet focuses on whole, nutrient-dense foods, in particular emphasizing:

- **Fruits and Vegetables:** These are rich sources of antioxidants, which are central compounds that inhibit oxidative stress. Antioxidants neutralize free radicals—molecules that can damage cells and contribute to chronic inflammation. Consuming a rainbow of colorful fruits and vegetables such as berries, oranges, and leafy greens ensures an intake of various antioxidants, like polyphenols, beta-carotene and lycopene, which each combat different types of oxidative stress and protect against inflammation.

- **Omega-3 Fatty Acids:** These essential fats are crucial in reducing inflammation and are potent anti-inflammatory warriors. EPA and DHA, two types of omega-3s found predominantly in fatty fish such as salmon, sardines and mackerel, are especially effective. They help reduce the production of inflammatory eicosanoids and cytokines. Plant-based sources like algae, flaxseeds, and chia seeds offer ALA, another type of omega-3 fatty acid, which the body partially converts to EPA and DHA.

- **Fiber:** High-fiber foods enhance the growth of health-promoting gut bacteria, which help manage the immune system and reduce inflammation by breaking down fiber into short-chain fatty acids, which in turn possess anti-inflammatory properties. Fiber helps regulate inflammation by reducing the permeability of the intestines and thus decreasing the chances of inflammation-causing substances entering the bloodstream. Sources of soluble fiber like oats, apples, and beans, as well as sources of insoluble fiber like whole grains and vegetables, are both beneficial. High-fiber foods such as dark-colored leafy greens, carrots, broccoli, whole grains, beans, and lentils all support the growth of beneficial gut bacteria.

- **Probiotics and Prebiotics:** Probiotics found in fermented foods like yogurt, kefir, kimchi and sauerkraut introduce beneficial bacteria into the digestive system. These bacteria contain live cultures that enhance gut health and can significantly lower systemic inflammation by improving the intestinal barrier, which prevents harmful substances from entering the bloodstream and triggering an immune response. Prebiotics found in foods like bananas, onions, and garlic feed these beneficial bacteria.

- **Herbs and Spices:** Many herbs and spices are loaded with anti-inflammatory compounds. For example, turmeric contains curcumin, a substance with powerful anti-inflammatory and antioxidant properties. Similarly, ginger and garlic offer bioactive molecules that suppress pro-inflammatory compounds produced by the body.

Adopting an anti-inflammatory diet in the real-world everyday life involves more than just choosing the right foods; it requires integrating these choices into a holistic lifestyle that includes regular exercise, stress management, and sufficient sleep—all of which play a significant role in controlling inflammation and profoundly reshaping your health. As you begin this dietary exploration, it's important to remember that diversity is crucial—incorporating a wide array of anti-inflammatory foods ensures a comprehensive array of nutrients, effectively keeping chronic inflammation in check and boosting your overall health and longevity.

Health Benefits of an Anti-Inflammatory Diet

Over the years, I've witnessed the profound impact that dietary choices have on reducing chronic inflammation and promoting overall well-being. An anti-inflammatory diet goes beyond mere health trends; it is a science-supported strategy that can profoundly improve your quality of life. This approach significantly mitigates the risk of various chronic diseases, bolsters mental health, promotes digestive wellness, and assists in effective weight management. So, what are the health benefits of an anti-inflammatory diet? There are numerous advantages to consider, and here are some of the most critical ones.

- **Reduced Risk of Chronic Diseases:** Chronic inflammation is a silent threat that contributes to major health conditions like heart disease, diabetes, arthritis, and even Alzheimer's disease. An anti-inflammatory diet combats this by incorporating foods rich in omega-3 fatty acids, antioxidants, and phytonutrients. For instance, the omega-3 fatty acids found in fatty fish like salmon and mackerel, or in plant sources like flaxseeds and chia seeds, are known for their ability to reduce the levels of inflammatory markers in the blood. These foods inhibit the production of inflammation-promoting substances like prostaglandins and leukotrienes, thus protecting cardiovascular health and enhancing joint mobility.

- **Enhanced Mental Health and Cognitive Function:** The relationship between diet and mental health is increasingly evident. Diets high in processed foods and sugars can exacerbate inflammation that may worsen symptoms of depression and anxiety. Conversely, foods rich in antioxidants—such as berries, dark chocolate, and leafy greens—and healthy fats, like those found in avocados and olive oil, not only fight inflammation but also support brain health. Through research these foods have been repeatedly linked to reductions in depressive symptoms and a lower risk of cognitive decline. An anti-inflammatory diet provides vital nutrients like polyphenols and flavonoids that protect the brain from oxidative stress and inflammation, thereby preserving cognitive functions.

- **Improved Digestive Health:** Gastrointestinal health can be significantly improved by adopting an anti-inflammatory diet. Inflammatory bowel diseases (IBD) such as Crohn's disease and ulcerative colitis respond well to diets high in fiber from whole grains and legumes, which foster a healthy gut microbiome. Fermented foods like kimchi, sauerkraut, and probiotic yogurts introduce beneficial bacteria into the gut, helping to maintain an optimal balance of gut flora, which is essential in reducing inflammation and enhancing digestive health.

- **Better Physical Fitness and Weight Management:** Inflammation is often linked with obesity and metabolic syndrome. An anti-inflammatory diet helps manage body weight by prioritizing whole, nutrient-dense foods over calorie-dense but nutritionally poor foods. Foods high in soluble fiber, such as broccoli, apples, and carrots, not only provide a prolonged feeling of fullness but also reduce the absorption of fats and improve blood sugar control, aiding in weight management and metabolic health.

- **Increased Longevity:** One of the most compelling benefits of an anti-inflammatory diet is its potential to extend lifespan. Chronic inflammation has been associated with accelerated aging and the onset of age-related diseases. By reducing inflammation, this diet helps preserve cellular function and delays aging processes. Regular consumption of anti-inflammatory foods can thus not only add years to your life but also life to your years, allowing you to enjoy a more active, fulfilling life.

In essence, the anti-inflammatory diet is a powerful tool for promoting long-term health, strength and an overall energy level. It is a way of eating that values quality, nutrition, and health benefits, making every meal an opportunity to nourish and heal your body. By embracing this diet, you invest in a future of enhanced health and increased well-being.

Inflammation Warriors

As previously discussed, an effective anti-inflammatory diet relies on a foundation of nutrient-dense foods that actively work to reduce systemic inflammation. To give you a clearer idea of how to nourish your body, here's a detailed list of essentials to regularly include in your diet, each playing a crucial role in fighting inflammation:

- **Monounsaturated Fats:** These fats, found in olive oil, avocados, and certain nuts, help reduce the risk of heart disease by lowering bad cholesterol levels and providing fats that are anti-inflammatory. The phenolic compounds in extra virgin olive oil, for instance, are effective in reducing inflammation.

- **Polyphenols:** Polyphenols such as flavonoids, resveratrol and curcumin help neutralize free radicals, inhibit pro-inflammatory transcription factors, leading to protective effects against many inflammation-caused chronic diseases. For example, flavonoid-rich foods like green tea, dark chocolate, and citrus fruits not only help in managing inflammation but also supports cardiovascular health and weight management. Resveratrol in grapes and curcumin in turmeric have also been extensively studied for their powerful anti-inflammatory properties.

- **Bioactive Compounds:** Spices and herbs like turmeric, ginger, garlic, and cinnamon are not only rich in flavor but also have impressive anti-inflammatory benefits. Ginger and garlic, for instance, contain compounds that inhibit the synthesis of pro-inflammatory cytokines in the body.

- **Selenium:** Selenium is a vital micronutrient that acts as a co-factor for antioxidant enzymes like glutathione peroxidase, which plays a key role in preventing cellular damage from free radicals. A selenium-rich diet is linked not only to reduced inflammation but also to enhanced immunity and lower rates of oxidative stress. Foods high in selenium include Brazil nuts, seafood like tuna and shrimp, and sunflower seeds, which make integrating selenium into your diet both easy and delicious.

- **Zinc:** Zinc is crucial for maintaining a robust immune system. It directly inhibits the inflammatory process by competing with inflammatory cytokines and reducing oxidative stress. Zinc is also essential for hormone production and can enhance skin health, which is often compromised by chronic inflammation. High-zinc foods include oysters, beef, spinach, and pumpkin seeds, offering a variety of choices for different dietary preferences.

- **Quercetin:** Quercetin is a powerful flavonoid known for its anti-inflammatory and antioxidant effects. It helps in reducing inflammation by inhibiting enzymes involved in the synthesis of inflammatory mediators and by scavenging free radicals. Regular intake of quercetin-rich foods such as apples, onions, and capers can help manage a range of inflammatory conditions, including chronic diseases like heart disease and asthma.

- **Anthocyanins:** These compounds not only give fruits and vegetables their vibrant red, purple, and blue hues but also are potent anti-inflammatory agents. They work by blocking inflammatory pathways and preventing the formation of inflammatory cytokines. Foods rich in anthocyanins, such as cherries, raspberries, blackberries, and blueberries, can be particularly beneficial for reducing the risk of cardiovascular disease and cancer.

- **Vitamin E:** Known for its antioxidant properties, vitamin E is essential in protecting the body from oxidative stress which can lead to chronic inflammation. It also plays a role in enhancing immune function and preventing clots, which can contribute to heart disease. Almonds, spinach, and sweet potatoes are excellent sources of vitamin E, making them a great addition to an anti-inflammatory diet.

- **Carotenoids:** These antioxidants are critical for neutralizing free radicals, reducing oxidative stress, and thereby diminishing inflammation. Beta-carotene, lutein, and lycopene are some types of carotenoids that have been shown to improve immune function and protect against the damaging effects of inflammation. Carrots, sweet potatoes, and spinach are all excellent sources.

- **Magnesium:** Magnesium has a calming effect on the nervous system and can counteract stress, which is a common trigger of inflammation. This mineral also plays a role in hundreds of biochemical reactions in the body, including those that regulate the immune response. Incorporating magnesium-rich foods like leafy greens, nuts, and whole grains can help maintain proper inflammatory responses and overall health.

- **Isoflavones:** Particularly beneficial for women, isoflavones mimic estrogen and can help balance hormones, which is often crucial in controlling inflammation-related conditions such as menopause symptoms and osteoporosis. Non-GMO and organic soy products like tofu and tempeh are rich in isoflavones and offer a plant-based protein source that supports overall health.

- **Vitamin K:** Beyond its well-known role in blood clotting, vitamin K also plays an essential role in regulating inflammatory responses. It helps in maintaining bone health by regulating calcium deposition, thus preventing inflammatory diseases such as osteoarthritis. Foods rich in vitamin K include kale, spinach, and broccoli.

- **Allicin:** Found in garlic, allicin is released when garlic is chopped or crushed. This compound has been shown to reduce inflammation by inhibiting the activation of inflammatory pathways in the body. Allicin also has antimicrobial properties, which can help prevent and reduce infections, often a hidden source of chronic inflammation.

- **Capsaicin:** Capsaicin in chili peppers provides pain relief by reducing substance P, a chemical that signals pain to the brain. It also has anti-inflammatory properties by decreasing the production of inflammatory cytokines. Adding moderate amounts of chili pepper to dishes can provide these benefits along with a spicy flavor.

- **Luteolin:** This flavonoid inhibits various inflammatory responses, including the production of inflammatory cytokines and enzymes. It's found in high amounts in celery, thyme, and green peppers, making it an easy addition to many meals for an anti-inflammatory boost.

- **Resistant Starch:** Resistant starch acts as a prebiotic, feeding good bacteria in the gut, which are vital for a healthy immune system and managing inflammation. Foods rich in resistant starch, such as green bananas, and cooked and cooled rice and potatoes, can help improve gut health and reduce systemic inflammation.

- **Pantothenic Acid (Vitamin B5):** This vitamin helps with energy metabolism and the synthesis of adrenal hormones, which are crucial for managing stress and inflammation. Mushrooms, avocados, and sunflower seeds are good sources and can easily be incorporated into various dishes.

- **Copper:** Copper not only helps maintain metabolic processes but also plays a key role in reducing symptoms of rheumatoid arthritis, a chronic inflammatory condition. Foods like sesame seeds, cashews, and soybeans are rich in copper and provide additional nutrients beneficial for overall health.

By incorporating these diverse components into your diet, you can effectively manage inflammation and improve your overall health. Each component offers unique benefits and, when combined, can significantly enhance the anti-inflammatory effects of your diet.

Foods to Eat and Foods to Avoid

Foods to Eat on an Anti-Inflammatory Diet

Category	Sub-category	Examples
Fruits	Berries	Blueberries, strawberries, raspberries, blackberries
	Citrus	Oranges, lemons, limes, grapefruits
	Tropical*	Açaí, papaya, pineapple, lychee, mamey, passion fruit, jackfruit, mango, kiwi
	Stone Fruits	Peaches, nectarines, plums, apricots
Vegetables	Leafy Greens	Spinach, kale, Swiss chard, collard greens
	Cruciferous	Broccoli, cauliflower, Brussels sprouts, cabbage
	Root	Sweet potatoes, carrots, beets, radishes
	Nightshades*	Bell peppers, tomatoes, eggplants, white potatoes
	Squashes	Butternut squash, acorn squash, spaghetti squash, zucchini
Whole Grains	Gluten-Free	Quinoa, brown rice, millet, buckwheat
	Others	Oats, whole wheat, barley, farro, teff
Healthy Fats	Nuts	Almonds, walnuts, cashews, pistachios, macadamia nuts
	Seeds	Flaxseeds, chia seeds, hemp seeds, pumpkin seeds
	Oils	Olive oil, avocado oil, flaxseed oil, coconut oil
Protein Sources	Legumes	Lentils, chickpeas, black beans, kidney beans
	Fish	Salmon, mackerel, sardines, anchovies, trout
	Poultry and Eggs	Organic chicken, turkey, pasture-raised eggs
Spices/Herbs	Spices	Turmeric, ginger, cinnamon, nutmeg, cardamom, black pepper, cayenne, cloves, fenugreek, allspice, bay leaves, ginseng
	Herbs	Basil, thyme, rosemary, parsley, cilantro, sage, oregano
Beverages	Teas	Green tea, herbal teas, black tea, white tea
	Other	Water, natural fruit juices*, vegetable juices, kombucha

* Should be consumed in moderation

Neutral Foods (Considered in Moderation)

Category	Sub-category	Examples
Red Meat	Grass-Fed and Organic	Grass-fed beef, lamb

Neutral Foods (Considered in Moderation)

Dairy	Grass-Fed and Organic	Organic high-fat dairy, such as cheese, kefir and unsweetened yogurt

Foods to Avoid on an Anti-Inflammatory Diet

Category	Sub-category	Examples
Refined Sugars	Sweeteners	Table sugar, corn syrup, high-fructose corn syrup
	Sweets	Candy, chocolate bars, ice cream, baked goods, cakes
Refined Carbs	Breads	White bread, bagels, croissants, muffins, pastries
	Snacks	Pretzels, crackers, chips, cookies, breakfast cereal
Unhealthy Fats	Trans Fats	Margarine, vegetable shortening, fried foods
	Saturated Fats	High-fat cuts of commercial meat, butter, cream
Processed Meats	All	Sausages, bacon, hot dogs, deli meats
Dairy	Processed	Processed cheese, ice cream, flavored yogurts
Additives	Preservatives	Sodium nitrate, monosodium glutamate (MSG)
	Artificial Colorants	Red 40, Yellow 5, Blue 1
Beverages	Alcoholic	Beer, wine, spirits
	Sugary Drinks	Soda, sweetened teas, energy drinks
Nightshades	Sensitive Individuals	Tomatoes, white potatoes, bell peppers, eggplants

Chapter 2: Preparing for Your Journey

Setting Up Your Kitchen for Success

Setting up your kitchen with these tools and staples ensures you're always ready to prepare meals that support an anti-inflammatory diet. As a seasoned nutritionist dedicated to anti-inflammatory practices, I can attest to the profound impact that a properly organized and equipped kitchen can have on the dietary success. Here are essential tips and strategies to optimize your kitchen setup, ensuring it supports your health goals seamlessly.

Essential Tools for Easy Meal Prep

To make meal preparation both enjoyable and effective, certain tools are indispensable in your kitchen. We recommend investing in some from the list below:

- **Versatile Blenders:** Ideal for making smoothies, soups, and sauces. Consider a high-powered model for versatility.

- **Diverse Knives:** A chef's knife, serrated knife, and paring knife cover most culinary tasks.

- **Sturdy Cutting Boards:** Opt for multiple boards to prevent cross-contamination, including bamboo or hardwood options.

- **Slow Cookers and Pressure Cookers:** Essential for hands-off cooking that preserves the nutrients in your foods.

- **Airtight Storage Containers:** Glass containers are preferable for storing prepped meals and avoiding plastic leach.

- **Mandoline Slicers and Spiralizers:** Excellent for creating uniform slices and noodles from vegetables.

- **Salad Spinners:** Wash and dry greens quickly to maintain freshness and ease of use in meals.

- **Spice Grinders:** Freshly ground spices like turmeric and black pepper enhance flavor and potency.

- **Juicers and Citrus Presses:** Extract pure juice from fruits and vegetables for hydration and anti-inflammatory benefits.

- **Digital Scales:** Ensure precise ingredient measurements, crucial for maintaining nutritional balance.

- **Parchment Paper:** Useful for non-stick baking and roasting without added oils and a great substitute for aluminium (foil) that can leach into food with cooking, especially when acidic juices and spice are added.

- **Cast Iron Skillets:** Excellent for searing and oven-finishing dishes, adding depth to flavors.

- **Food Processors:** Quickly chop, slice, dice, and blend ingredients for salsas, dips, and more.

- **Immersion Blenders:** Perfect for pureeing soups and sauces directly in the pot.

Pantry Staples for an Anti-Inflammatory Diet

Stocking your pantry with the right ingredients is key to maintaining an anti-inflammatory diet and stress-free meal planning. Below are some of the essentials to get you started:

- **Spices and Herbs:** Stock up on anti-inflammatory staples like turmeric, ginger, garlic, and black pepper. Add fresh herbs like basil, parsley, and cilantro to elevate the flavors in your dishes.

- **Whole Grains:** Incorporate a mix of grains such as quinoa, wild rice, farro, bulgur, amaranth, and teff, which are excellent for their anti-inflammatory properties and versatility in recipes.

- **Nuts and Seeds:** Beyond flax and chia, consider hemp seeds, walnuts, almonds, and pumpkin seeds for their healthy fats and anti-inflammatory properties. Make sure they are raw and unsalted to get the most benefits.

- **Legumes:** Broaden your range with varieties like navy beans, red lentils, and green peas, perfect for adding texture and protein to any meal. If possible, buy organic in dry form or in BPA-free cans.

- **Healthy Oils:** Keep a selection of cold-pressed oils like olive oil, avocado oil, and flaxseed oil, ideal for dressing salads or low-heat cooking.

- **Acidic Elements:** Apple cider vinegar and tamari sauce can add flavor to dishes while promoting a healthy pH balance and fighting inflammation.

- **Natural Sweeteners:** Opt for raw unpasteurized honey or pure maple syrup to sweeten dishes without adding refined sugar.

- **Fermented Foods:** Include options like sauerkraut, kimchi, and kefir, which promote gut health and reduce inflammation.

- **Nutritional Powders and Superfoods:** Consider adding powders such as beet, spirulina, maca, chaga mushrooms or green matcha, which can be easily integrated into smoothies for an extra nutrient kick. Incorporate goji berries, cacao nibs for their powerful antioxidant properties.

- **Herbal Teas:** Stock up on green tea, ginger tea, and turmeric tea and others; these are excellent for their anti-inflammatory effects.

- **Dried Fruits:** Small amounts of unsweetened dried cranberries, apricots, and dates can be great for adding natural sweetness to meals and snacks.

- **Canned Goods:** Look for BPA-free cans and low-sodium versions of salmon, sardines, tomatoes, and coconut milk for quick additions to meals.

Shopping and Budget Tips for Beginners

Adopting an anti-inflammatory diet doesn't have to break the bank. Here are some smart and easy strategies to start:

- **Wholesale and Bulk Purchases:** Buying staples like nuts, seeds, and whole grains in bulk can reduce costs significantly. For instance, purchasing bulk organic quinoa and storing it in airtight containers can be cost-effective and ensure you always have a quick-cooking grain available.

- **Buy Frozen:** Keep a variety of frozen mixed berries, veggies and dark leafy greens for quick smoothies or stir-fries.

- **Freeze To Preserve Freshness:** Freeze anti-inflammatory herbs in olive oil in ice cube trays, and store sliced breads and pastries in the freezer to avoid waste. Same goes for fresh ginger and turmeric roots; by freezing them you can grate them into dishes without sacrificing freshness.

- **Seasonal Produce:** Focus on buying fruits and vegetables when they are in season. Explore farmers' markets for fresh produce, not only is this more economical, but seasonal produce also tends to be higher in nutrients. For example, buying strawberries during peak season ensures better flavor and antioxidant content.

- **Plan Your Meals:** Weekly meal planning reduces impulse buys and ensures you use what you buy, minimizing waste.

- **Subscription Services:** Consider subscribing to a grocery delivery service that focuses on whole foods to simplify shopping and introduce variety.

Understanding Food Labels

Navigating food labels is a critical skill for anyone committed to an anti-inflammatory diet. Being a passionate anti-inflammatory nutritionist for many years, I've guided my clients, friends and family members through the nuances of packaged foods to help them avoid hidden inflammatory triggers. This detailed guide will expand your understanding of food labels, ensuring you make the healthiest choices for reducing inflammation.

Deep Diving into Ingredients and Nutritional Facts

Understanding food labels is key with everyday grocery shopping and begins with a thorough analysis of ingredients and nutritional content, focusing on transparency and health implications. Over time this habit will help you make healthier eating choices and identify nutrient-dense foods for a healthy diet.

- **Whole and Simple Ingredients:** Opt for products with simple, recognizable ingredients. Avoid foods with long lists of additives or unfamiliar terms, as these are often highly processed.

- **Fats and Oils:** Identify heart-healthy fats essential for an anti-inflammatory diet, such as olive oil, coconut oil, and those in nuts and seeds. Steer clear of hydrogenated oils, seed oils such as canola and sunflower oils and trans fats, which are pro-inflammatory.

- **Sugars and Sweeteners:** Sugars are major inflammatory agents. Beyond the obvious (sugar, high fructose corn syrup), be wary of anhydrous dextrose, fruit juice concentrates, maltose, dextrin, and syrup names. Opt for natural sweeteners like honey or maple syrup in moderation.

- **Protein Sources:** Look for lean, unprocessed protein sources, organic and pasture-raised if possible. Be cautious of processed meats, which often contain nitrates and high levels of sodium.

- **Fiber Content:** High fiber content is beneficial for managing inflammation. Foods rich in fiber, like whole grains, leafy greens and vegetables, should be featured prominently in daily meals.

○ **Sodium and Salt:** High sodium can exacerbate inflammation, especially in individuals with hypertension or autoimmune diseases. Opt for low-sodium versions of products, particularly in canned and boxed foods.

Unmasking Hidden Sources of Inflammation

For those new to an anti-inflammatory diet, understanding and identifying hidden sources of inflammation in packaged foods is crucial. Hidden inflammatory ingredients can sabotage your anti-inflammatory diet without you even knowing.

This table provides a foundational understanding of the ingredients to avoid or limit in your diet and offers practical alternatives that support an anti-inflammatory lifestyle. For those just starting on this path, focusing on whole unprocessed foods, is always a beneficial strategy. By making mindful choices and understanding the reasons behind them, you can effectively manage inflammation through your diet.

Common Sources of Inflammation	Often Found In...	Reasons For Inflammation	Swap For...
Artificial Additives (including artificial flavors, colors, and enhancers such as monosodium glutamate (MSG), Yellow #5, Red #40, Blue #1)	Processed snacks (potato chips, flavored crackers), candies (gummies, hard candy), soft drinks, frozen dinners, fast food burgers, instant noodles, microwave popcorn, flavored yogurt, packaged sauces (e.g., BBQ sauce), artificially colored ice creams	Artificial additives disrupt gut microbiota, weaken the immune system, and increase inflammation in the digestive tract, which may trigger bloating, gas, abdominal pain, and irritable bowel syndrome (IBS). Artificial colors like Red #40 and Yellow #5 have been linked to hyperactivity in children and allergic reactions. Chronic exposure can also worsen conditions like asthma and migraines.	Snacks labeled "no artificial additives," homemade popcorn, organic or naturally flavored snacks, fresh fruit
Preservatives (BHT, BHA, sodium benzoate, potassium sorbate, sulfites)	Breakfast cereals (cornflakes, rice krispies), chips (corn chips, potato chips), canned vegetables, shelf-stable baked goods (cookies, cupcakes), processed meats (hot dogs, sausages, deli meats), frozen meals, soft drinks, boxed cake mixes, bottled sauces (ketchup, BBQ sauce), packaged cheeses, dried fruits (with added sulfites)	Preservatives like BHT and BHA generate reactive oxygen species (free radicals) that contribute to cellular damage and chronic inflammation, which accelerates aging and increases the risk of cancer. Sulfites can trigger asthma and allergies in sensitive individuals, while sodium benzoate has been linked to hyperactivity and oxidative stress, causing damage to cell membranes and DNA over time.	Organic cereals and snacks without preservatives, fresh baked goods, nitrate-free meats, homemade condiments, dried fruits without preservatives

Common Sources of Inflammation	Often Found In...	Reasons For Inflammation	Swap For...
Refined Carbohydrates (enriched flour, high fructose corn syrup, maltodextrin, dextrose)	White bread, pasta, pastries (donuts, danishes), cakes (boxed cake mixes, store-bought cakes), cookies (Oreos, Chips Ahoy), crackers, instant mashed potatoes, pancakes, waffles, pretzels, breakfast bars, cereal bars, sugary cereals (Frosted Flakes, Cap'n Crunch), processed pizza dough	Refined carbohydrates cause rapid spikes in blood sugar, which promote insulin resistance and type 2 diabetes. This leads to chronic low-grade inflammation, which is associated with increased risk of heart disease, obesity, and metabolic syndrome. These foods also disrupt gut health by feeding bad bacteria, contributing to leaky gut syndrome, which worsens autoimmune conditions like rheumatoid arthritis and psoriasis.	Whole grain bread, whole wheat pasta, rice pasta, lentil pasta, sprouted grain bread, quinoa, sweet potatoes, steel-cut oats
Omega-6 Fatty Acids (soybean oil, corn oil, safflower oil, sunflower oil, vegetable oil)	Vegetable oils (soybean, corn, safflower oil), margarine, processed salad dressings, mayonnaise, fried foods (French fries, fried chicken), snack foods (potato chips, corn chips), processed peanut butter, pizza, microwave popcorn, packaged baked goods	Excessive omega-6 fatty acids stimulate the production of pro-inflammatory molecules like cytokines and eicosanoids, which aggravate conditions such as arthritis, cardiovascular disease, and chronic pain. An imbalanced ratio of omega-6 to omega-3 can exacerbate skin conditions like eczema and acne, as well as lead to mood disorders like depression and anxiety due to brain inflammation.	Olive oil, flaxseed oil, avocado oil, walnut oil, homemade salad dressings with olive oil, raw or lightly roasted nuts
Gluten (wheat, barley, rye, malt, wheat protein, semolina)	Breads (bagels, rolls), pastas, cereals, crackers (wheat crackers), pizza, pancakes, cookies, cakes, pastries, couscous, some soups (as a thickener), soy sauce, beer	Gluten triggers an immune response in the gut for individuals with celiac disease and non-celiac gluten sensitivity, leading to inflammation, bloating, gas, and diarrhea. Long-term inflammation in the gut can cause leaky gut, allowing toxins and undigested proteins to enter the bloodstream, which exacerbates autoimmune diseases, joint pain, skin rashes, and neurological issues like brain fog and migraines.	Gluten-free breads and pastas (rice, almond flour, or chickpea-based), gluten-free crackers, almond flour pancakes, tamari (gluten-free soy sauce), quinoa, millet, brown rice
Dairy (lactose, casein,	Milk, cheese (cheddar, mozzarella, parmesan), yogurt, ice cream, butter, cream cheese,	Dairy products are high in hormones and saturated fats, which can cause inflammation,	Almond milk, coconut yogurt, cashew cheese, oat

Common Sources of Inflammation	Often Found In...	Reasons For Inflammation	Swap For...
whey protein, milk solids)	whipped cream, cream-based sauces (Alfredo sauce), commercial smoothies, protein shakes, chocolate, baked goods (cakes, cookies), pizza, mac & cheese	especially in people who are lactose intolerant or sensitive to casein. Symptoms include bloating, gas, diarrhea, and constipation. Chronic dairy consumption can exacerbate acne, sinus congestion, and increase mucus production. Inflammatory reactions can worsen conditions like IBS, asthma, joint pain, and certain autoimmune disorders such as Hashimoto's thyroiditis and lupus.	milk, plant-based creamers, nutritional yeast, dairy-free ice creams
Emulsifiers and Thickeners (carrageenan, xanthan gum, guar gum, polysorbates, lecithin, mono- and diglycerides)	Ice cream (store-bought, low-fat versions), salad dressings (ranch, Caesar), sauces (store-bought marinara, Alfredo), non-dairy milks (almond, soy, oat milk), mayonnaise, whipped toppings, peanut butter, jelly, chocolate milk, energy bars, frozen desserts, dips (hummus, spinach dip)	Emulsifiers disrupt the gut barrier, contributing to intestinal inflammation and worsening conditions like inflammatory bowel disease (IBD) and Crohn's disease. They also promote dysbiosis by feeding harmful gut bacteria, which can lead to bloating, gas, diarrhea, and fatigue. In the long term, chronic inflammation from emulsifiers may increase the risk of metabolic syndrome and obesity.	Natural thickeners like agar, pectin-based sauces, chia seed puddings, full-fat natural dairy, homemade almond milk, homemade nut butters
High Fructose Corn Syrup (HFCS, corn syrup, fructose, glucose syrup)	Sodas, sweetened iced teas, fruit-flavored drinks, sports drinks, flavored yogurts, candy bars, fruit snacks, ketchup, BBQ sauce, salad dressings, packaged cakes (Twinkies, Little Debbie), breakfast cereals (Froot Loops, Frosted Flakes), granola bars, pancake syrup	High fructose corn syrup promotes the accumulation of visceral fat, which increases inflammation in the liver, leading to non-alcoholic fatty liver disease (NAFLD). It also triggers an inflammatory response in fat cells, causing insulin resistance, diabetes, and obesity. HFCS increases the production of inflammatory cytokines, promoting systemic inflammation and increasing the risk of heart disease and high blood pressure.	Beverages sweetened with honey or maple syrup, homemade fruit sauces, stevia or monk fruit sweeteners, plain yogurt with fresh fruit, whole fruit smoothies
Trans Fats (partially hydrogenated oils,	Fried foods (French fries, chicken nuggets, fried fish), packaged cookies (Oreos, Chips Ahoy),	Trans fats contribute to oxidative stress and systemic inflammation, damaging blood vessels and	Homemade baked goods using coconut oil or real

Common Sources of Inflammation	Often Found In…	Reasons For Inflammation	Swap For...
shortening, margarine)	cakes (store-bought frosted cakes, cupcakes), frozen pizza, margarine, shortening, microwave popcorn, non-dairy coffee creamers, frozen pies, canned frosting, refrigerated dough (biscuits, cinnamon rolls)	increasing the risk of cardiovascular disease, stroke, and high cholesterol. They also promote the production of inflammatory cytokines, worsening conditions like atherosclerosis, arthritis, and diabetes. Ingesting trans fats may also contribute to weight gain and belly fat accumulation, which further exacerbates inflammatory responses.	butter, air-fried or oven-baked snacks, avocado, nuts, butter or ghee
Artificial Sweeteners (aspartame, sucralose, saccharin, acesulfame potassium, sorbitol)	Diet sodas, sugar-free gum, flavored water, light yogurt, sugar-free ice cream, protein bars, meal replacement shakes, sugar-free candy, diet desserts, sugar-free coffee sweeteners, low-calorie snacks	Artificial sweeteners can disrupt the gut microbiome, leading to glucose intolerance and metabolic syndrome. Aspartame has been linked to increased oxidative stress and inflammation in the brain, which may worsen neurological conditions like migraines, depression, and multiple sclerosis (MS). Overconsumption of artificial sweeteners can also promote insulin resistance, obesity, and increased cravings for sugary foods, fueling a vicious cycle of inflammation.	Snacks sweetened with stevia or small amounts of raw honey, whole fruit, maple syrup, homemade desserts with natural sweeteners
Nitrites/Nitrates (sodium nitrite, sodium nitrate, potassium nitrate)	Processed meats (bacon, ham, salami, sausages, deli meats), hot dogs, jerky, cured meats (pepperoni, corned beef), canned meats (spam), frozen dinners with meat, packaged lunch kits, smoked fish, pre-cooked sausages	Nitrites and nitrates form reactive nitrogen species in the body, which cause oxidative stress and damage cells and tissues, leading to chronic inflammation. Regular consumption of processed meats increases the risk of colorectal cancer, cardiovascular disease, and hypertension due to the inflammatory effects. Nitrites also worsen inflammation in the gastrointestinal tract, which may exacerbate digestive issues and increase the risk of ulcers.	Freshly prepared meats, nitrate-free processed meats, homemade sausages, fresh seafood, uncured bacon

Common Sources of Inflammation	Often Found In...	Reasons For Inflammation	Swap For...
Alcohol (ethanol, ethyl alcohol, alcohol-containing flavor extracts)	Beer, wine, spirits (vodka, rum, whiskey), cocktails, liqueur-based desserts (rum cake, tiramisu), alcohol-flavored marinades, sauces made with alcohol (vodka sauce, beer-battered foods), vanilla extract, some cough syrups	Alcohol increases gut permeability, allowing toxins and bacteria to enter the bloodstream, triggering systemic inflammation. It also promotes oxidative stress in the liver, leading to fatty liver disease and cirrhosis. Chronic alcohol consumption is linked to inflammatory conditions like gastritis, pancreatitis, liver disease, and increased risk of certain cancers. Additionally, alcohol disrupts the immune system and may aggravate autoimmune diseases like lupus and rheumatoid arthritis.	Vanilla extract without alcohol, alcohol-free desserts, kombucha, mocktails, herbal teas

Chapter 3: Breakfast

Deluxe Smoked Salmon Avocado Toast

Prep Time: 15 min

Cook Time: 5 min

Serves: 2

Ingredients

- 2 slices of gluten-free whole grain bread
- 1 large ripe avocado
- 4 oz smoked salmon
- 2 eggs
- 1 tbsp white vinegar
- Fresh dill for garnish
- Freshly cracked black pepper
- Pinch of sea salt
- 1 tsp of capers for topping (optional)

Directions

1. Halve the avocado, remove the pit, and scoop out the flesh into a bowl. Mash it with a fork, season with salt and pepper, and set aside.

2. Toast gluten-free bread slices until golden and crispy.

3. Heat a pot of water to a gentle simmer, add white vinegar, and carefully slide the eggs into the water. Poach for 3-4 minutes, then remove with a slotted spoon and drain.

4. Spread the mashed avocado on the toasted bread, add smoked salmon slices, and top each with a poached egg. Garnish with dill and capers, if using.

Nutritional Information: Calories: 400, Protein: 25g, Carbohydrates: 30g, Fat: 22g, Fiber: 7g, Cholesterol: 186mg, Sodium: 600mg

Savory Breakfast Quinoa Bowl

Prep Time: 10 min

Cook Time: 20 min

Serves: 4

Ingredients

- 1 cup quinoa, rinsed
- 2 cups water
- 1 tbsp olive oil
- 4 cloves garlic, minced
- 4 cups mixed greens (such as kale, spinach, and Swiss chard), chopped
- 1 ripe avocado, sliced
- 4 tbsp nutritional yeast
- Salt and pepper to taste

Directions

1. In a medium saucepan, combine quinoa and water. Bring to a boil, then reduce heat to low, cover, and simmer for about 15 minutes, or until the water is absorbed and the quinoa is tender.

2. While the quinoa cooks, heat the olive oil in a large skillet over medium heat. Add the garlic and sauté for 1 minute until fragrant.

3. Add the mixed greens to the skillet and sauté for about 5 minutes, or until wilted. Season with salt and pepper to taste.

4. Divide the cooked quinoa among four bowls. Top each bowl with sautéed greens and sliced avocado. Sprinkle each bowl with 1 tablespoon of nutritional yeast before serving.

Nutritional Information: Calories: 280, Protein: 10g, Carbohydrates: 31g, Fat: 14g, Fiber: 7g, Cholesterol: 0mg, Sodium: 40mg

Spinach and Mushroom Breakfast Hash

Ingredients

- 2 large sweet potatoes, peeled and diced
- 1 tbsp olive oil
- 1 red onion, diced
- 2 cloves garlic, minced
- 1 bell pepper, diced
- 8 oz mushrooms, sliced
- 4 cups fresh spinach
- 1 tsp smoked paprika
- Salt and black pepper to taste
- 4 eggs (optional)

 Prep Time: 15 min

 Cook Time: 20 min

 Serves: 4

Directions

1. Heat the olive oil in a large skillet over medium heat. Add the sweet potatoes and sauté for about 10 minutes, or until they begin to soften.

2. Add the onion, garlic, and bell pepper to the skillet. Cook for an additional 5 minutes until the onion is translucent.

3. Stir in the mushrooms and smoked paprika, and cook for another 5 minutes until the mushrooms have softened.

4. Add the spinach and cook until it wilts, about 2 minutes. Season with salt and pepper to taste.

5. Optional: In a separate pan, fry or poach eggs to your liking and serve on top of the hash for added protein.

Nutritional Information: Calories: 200, Protein: 6g, Carbohydrates: 30g, Fat: 7g, Fiber: 5g, Cholesterol: 0mg, Sodium: 75mg

Chia and Pumpkin Seed Pudding

Ingredients

- 1/4 cup chia seeds
- 1 cup unsweetened almond milk
- 1 cup coconut milk
- 2 tbsp pure maple syrup
- 1/2 tsp vanilla extract
- 1/4 cup pumpkin seeds
- Fresh berries or a sprinkle of cinnamon powder (optional toppings)

 Prep Time: 10 min

Cook Time: 4 hours

Serves: 4

Directions

1. In a medium bowl, combine chia seeds, almond milk, coconut milk, maple syrup, and vanilla extract. Stir well to mix.

2. Cover the bowl with a lid or plastic wrap and refrigerate for at least 4 hours, or overnight, until the mixture thickens and becomes gelatinous.

3. Toast the pumpkin seeds in a dry skillet over medium heat for about 3-5 minutes, stirring frequently until they are lightly browned and fragrant.

4. Once the pudding has set, stir it well and divide it into four servings.

5. Top each serving with toasted pumpkin seeds and, if desired, fresh berries or a sprinkle of cinnamon before serving.

Nutritional Information: Calories: 220, Protein: 6g, Carbohydrates: 18g, Fat: 15g, Fiber: 5g, Cholesterol: 0mg, Sodium: 45mg

Almond Flour Pancakes with Blueberries

Ingredients

- 2 cups almond flour
- 1 tsp baking powder
- 1/4 tsp salt
- 2 eggs
- 1/2 cup unsweetened almond milk
- 1 tbsp maple syrup (optional)
- 1 tsp vanilla extract
- 1/2 cup fresh blueberries
- Coconut oil or butter for cooking

 Prep Time: 10 min   Cook Time: 15 min   Serves: 4

Directions

1. In a large bowl, whisk together almond flour, baking powder, and salt.
2. In another bowl, beat the eggs and then mix in the almond milk, maple syrup, and vanilla extract.
3. Pour the wet ingredients into the dry ingredients and stir until just combined.
4. Fold in the blueberries gently to avoid breaking them.
5. Heat a skillet over medium heat and grease lightly with coconut oil or butter.
6. Pour about 1/4 cup of batter for each pancake onto the hot skillet. Cook for about 2-3 minutes on each side or until golden brown and cooked through.
7. Serve hot with additional blueberries and maple syrup if desired.

Nutritional Information: Calories: 345, Protein: 12g, Carbohydrates: 20g, Fat: 25g, Fiber: 6g, Cholesterol: 93mg, Sodium: 300mg

Good For You Hummus Toast

Ingredients

- 4 slices of gluten-free bread
- 4 eggs
- 1 ripe avocado
- 1 small cucumber, thinly sliced
- 1/2 cup hummus
- Salt and pepper to taste
- Fresh dill or parsley for garnish (optional)

 Prep Time: 10 min   Cook Time: 5 min   Serves: 4

Directions

1. Toast the gluten-free bread slices until golden and crispy.
2. While the bread is toasting, fry or poach the eggs to your preferred doneness.
3. Spread each slice of toasted bread with a generous layer of hummus.
4. Mash the avocado and spread it evenly over the hummus.
5. Arrange the cucumber slices over the avocado.
6. Top each slice with a cooked egg. Season with salt and pepper, and garnish with fresh herbs if desired.

Nutritional Information: Calories: 300, Protein: 12g, Carbohydrates: 20g, Fat: 20g, Fiber: 6g, Cholesterol: 164mg, Sodium: 320mg

Zucchini and Red Pepper Frittata

Ingredients

- 6 large eggs
- 1 medium zucchini, thinly sliced
- 1 red bell pepper, diced
- 1 small onion, diced
- 2 tbsp olive oil
- 1/2 tsp salt
- 1/4 tsp black pepper
- 4 slices of gluten-free bread
- Fresh herbs (such as parsley or basil) for garnish (optional)

Prep Time: 15 min

Cook Time: 20 min

Serves: 4

Directions

1. Preheat your oven to 350°F (175°C).

2. In a medium skillet, heat the olive oil over medium heat. Add the onions and sauté until translucent, about 5 minutes.

3. Add the red bell pepper and zucchini to the skillet and sauté for an additional 5 minutes, until the vegetables are just tender.

4. In a large bowl, whisk the eggs with salt and pepper. Pour the egg mixture over the vegetables in the skillet. Cook for about 2-3 minutes until the edges begin to set.

5. Transfer the skillet to the oven and bake for 10-15 minutes, or until the frittata is fully set and lightly golden on top.

6. Toast the gluten-free bread slices until golden and crisp.

7. Serve the frittata with a slice of toasted gluten-free bread, and optionally garnish with fresh herbs.

Nutritional Information: Calories: 280, Protein: 14g, Carbohydrates: 18g, Fat: 17g, Fiber: 3g, Cholesterol: 370mg, Sodium: 430mg

Banana Nut Pancakes

Ingredients

- 1 cup rolled oats
- 1 ripe banana, mashed
- 1 cup almond milk
- 1 egg
- 1/2 tsp cinnamon powder
- 1/2 cup walnuts, chopped
- 1 tsp baking powder
- 1 tbsp honey (optional for sweetness)
- Coconut oil, for cooking

Prep Time: 10 min

Cook Time: 15 min

Serves: 4

Directions

1. In a blender, combine the rolled oats, mashed banana, almond milk, egg, cinnamon, and baking powder. Blend until smooth.

2. Stir in the chopped walnuts by hand.

3. Heat a skillet over medium heat and add a little coconut oil.

4. Pour about 1/4 cup of batter for each pancake onto the hot skillet. Cook for about 2-3 minutes on each side, or until pancakes are golden brown and cooked through.

5. Serve warm with a drizzle of honey if desired.

Nutritional Information: Calories: 280, Protein: 8g, Carbohydrates: 34g, Fat: 14g, Fiber: 5g, Cholesterol: 47mg, Sodium: 135mg

Kale and Sweet Potato Breakfast Tacos

Ingredients

- 2 medium sweet potatoes, peeled and diced
- 1 tbsp olive oil
- Salt and pepper to taste
- 1 bunch kale, stems removed and leaves chopped
- 1 tsp smoked paprika
- 8 small corn tortillas
- 1/2 cup chopped red onion
- 1 avocado, sliced
- Hot sauce or salsa for serving (optional)

Prep Time: 15 min

Cook Time: 20 min

Serves: 4

Directions

1. Preheat the oven to 400°F (200°C). Toss the diced sweet potatoes with olive oil, salt, and pepper. Spread them on a baking sheet and roast for 20 minutes, or until tender and golden.

2. While the sweet potatoes are roasting, heat a large skillet over medium heat. Add the chopped kale and a splash of water. Cook until the kale is wilted and tender, about 5-7 minutes. Season with smoked paprika, salt, and pepper.

3. Warm the corn tortillas in a dry skillet over medium heat or directly over a flame for a few seconds on each side until they are heated through.

4. Divide the roasted sweet potatoes and sautéed kale among the warmed tortillas. Top each taco with red onion slices and avocado.

5. Serve immediately, with optional hot sauce or salsa on the side.

Nutritional Information: Calories: 290, Protein: 5g, Carbohydrates: 45g, Fat: 11g, Fiber: 8g, Cholesterol: 0mg, Sodium: 75mg

Zucchini and Carrot Fritters

Ingredients

- 2 medium zucchinis, grated
- 2 medium carrots, grated
- 1/2 cup almond flour
- 2 large eggs, beaten
- 1 tsp garlic powder
- Salt and pepper to taste
- 4 tbsp avocado or olive oil
- 4 slices of gluten-free bread
- Fresh parsley or dill for garnish (optional)

Prep Time: 20 min

Cook Time: 10 min

Serves: 4

Directions

1. Place the grated zucchini in a colander, sprinkle with salt, and let it sit for 10 minutes. Squeeze out excess moisture using a clean towel.

2. In a large bowl, mix together the squeezed zucchini, grated carrots, almond flour, eggs, garlic powder, and season with salt and pepper.

3. Heat the olive oil in a large skillet over medium heat.

4. Form the vegetable mixture into small patties and fry in the skillet for about 4-5 minutes on each side, until golden brown and crispy.

5. Toast the gluten-free bread slices.

6. Serve the fritters on the toasted gluten-free bread, garnished with fresh herbs if desired.

Nutritional Information: Calories: 320, Protein: 8g, Carbohydrates: 23g, Fat: 23g, Fiber: 5g, Cholesterol: 93mg, Sodium: 320mg

Tempeh Bacon Lettuce Tomato Sandwich

Ingredients

- 8 oz tempeh, sliced into thin strips
- 2 tbsp soy sauce (or tamari for gluten-free option)
- 1 tbsp maple syrup
- 1 tsp smoked paprika
- 1/2 tsp garlic powder
- 1/2 tsp black pepper
- 1 tbsp olive oil
- 8 slices of whole grain bread (or gluten-free bread)
- 4 lettuce leaves
- 1 large tomato, sliced
- Vegan mayonnaise (optional)

Prep Time: 15 min

Cook Time: 10 min

Serves: 4

Directions

1. In a small bowl, mix the soy sauce, maple syrup, smoked paprika, garlic powder, and black pepper to create a marinade. Add the tempeh slices to the marinade, ensuring each piece is well-coated. Let sit for 10 minutes.

2. Heat olive oil in a skillet over medium heat. Add the marinated tempeh slices and cook for about 5 minutes on each side, or until crispy and browned.

3. Toast the bread slices until golden.

4. Assemble the sandwiches by spreading vegan mayonnaise (if using) on one side of each toasted bread slice, then layering a lettuce leaf, two or three slices of tomato, and a few pieces of the cooked tempeh bacon.

5. Close the sandwiches with the remaining slices of toasted bread and serve immediately.

Nutritional Information: Calories: 330, Protein: 19g, Carbohydrates: 35g, Fat: 13g, Fiber: 6g, Cholesterol: 0mg, Sodium: 620mg

Pear and Banana Wraps

Ingredients

- 4 whole grain or gluten-free tortillas
- 1/2 cup almond butter
- 2 ripe pears, thinly sliced
- 2 bananas, thinly sliced
- 2 tbsp honey (optional)

Prep Time: 10 min

Cook Time: 0 min

Serves: 4

Directions

1. Lay each tortilla flat on a clean surface.

2. Spread about 2 tablespoons of almond butter evenly over each tortilla.

3. Arrange the pear and banana slices over the almond butter on each tortilla.

4. Drizzle honey over the fruit if using, then roll up the tortillas tightly.

5. Cut each wrap in half before serving.

Nutritional Information: Calories: 350, Protein: 8g, Carbohydrates: 50g, Fat: 16g, Fiber: 7g, Cholesterol: 0mg, Sodium: 200mg

Cauliflower Breakfast Hash Browns

Ingredients

- 1 large head of cauliflower, grated
- 1 small onion, finely chopped
- 2 cloves garlic, minced
- 2 eggs, beaten
- 1/4 cup almond flour
- 1/2 tsp sea salt
- 1/4 tsp black pepper
- 2 tbsp olive oil for frying

 Prep Time: 15 min

 Cook Time: 15 min

 Serves: 4

Directions

1. In a large bowl, combine the grated cauliflower, onion, garlic, eggs, almond flour, salt, and pepper. Mix well until everything is evenly incorporated.

2. Heat the olive oil in a large skillet over medium heat. Scoop about 1/4 cup of the cauliflower mixture into the pan, flattening it into a hash brown shape.

3. Cook for about 7-8 minutes on each side or until golden brown and crispy. Repeat with the remaining mixture.

4. Drain the hash browns on paper towels to remove excess oil before serving.

Nutritional Information: Calories: 180, Protein: 7g, Carbohydrates: 14g, Fat: 11g, Fiber: 5g, Cholesterol: 93mg, Sodium: 320mg

Breakfast Apple Bake

Ingredients

- 2 cups rolled oats
- 1 large apple, peeled and diced
- 1/2 cup walnuts, chopped
- 1/3 cup raisins
- 2 cups almond milk
- 2 tbsp honey or maple syrup
- 1 tsp cinnamon powder
- 1/2 tsp nutmeg powder
- 1 tsp vanilla extract
- Pinch of salt

 Prep Time: 10 min

 Cook Time: 35 min

 Serves: 4

Directions

1. Preheat the oven to 375°F (190°C) and grease an 8-inch baking dish.

2. In a large bowl, mix together the oats, diced apple, walnuts, raisins, cinnamon, nutmeg, and salt.

3. In a separate bowl, whisk together the almond milk, honey (or maple syrup), and vanilla extract.

4. Pour the liquid mixture over the oat mixture and stir to combine. Transfer the mixture to the prepared baking dish.

5. Bake in the preheated oven for 35 minutes, or until the top is golden brown and the liquid has been absorbed.

Nutritional Information: Calories: 340, Protein: 8g, Carbohydrates: 50g, Fat: 12g, Fiber: 6g, Cholesterol: 0mg, Sodium: 80mg.

Veggie Egg Muffins

Ingredients

- 6 large eggs
- 1/2 cup almond milk (or organic dairy milk)
- 1 cup chopped broccoli
- 1 cup fresh spinach, chopped
- 1/2 cup diced red bell pepper
- 1/4 tsp salt
- 1/4 tsp black pepper
- 1/2 cup shredded cheese (optional or omit for dairy-free option)

 Prep Time: 15 min

 Cook Time: 20 min

 Serves: 6

Directions

1. Preheat the oven to 375°F (190°C) and grease a 12-cup muffin pan or line with muffin liners.
2. In a large bowl, whisk together eggs and milk until well combined. Season with salt and pepper.
3. Stir in the chopped broccoli, spinach, bell peppers, and cheese (if using) into the egg mixture.
4. Divide the mixture evenly among the muffin cups, filling each about 3/4 full.
5. Bake in the preheated oven for 20 minutes, or until the muffins are set in the center and lightly golden on top.

Nutritional Information: Calories: 110, Protein: 9g, Carbohydrates: 4g, Fat: 7g, Fiber: 1g, Cholesterol: 190mg, Sodium: 220mg

Cinnamon Apple Quinoa Breakfast Bowl

Ingredients

- 1 cup quinoa, rinsed
- 2 cups water
- 2 medium apples, diced
- 2 tbsp maple syrup
- 1 tsp cinnamon powder
- 1/4 cup chopped walnuts
- 1/4 cup raisins
- Pinch of salt
- Greek yogurt, almond milk, additional maple syrup for drizzling (optional toppings)

 Prep Time: 10 min

 Cook Time: 20 min

 Serves: 4

Directions

1. In a medium saucepan, combine the quinoa and water. Bring to a boil over medium heat.
2. Reduce the heat to low, cover, and simmer for 15-20 minutes, or until the quinoa is cooked and the water is absorbed.
3. While the quinoa is cooking, heat a skillet over medium heat. Add the diced apples, maple syrup, and cinnamon. Cook for 5-7 minutes, or until the apples are soft and caramelized.
4. Once the quinoa is cooked, fluff it with a fork and divide it among serving bowls. Top each bowl with the cooked apples, chopped walnuts, and raisins.
5. Serve hot, optionally drizzling with additional maple syrup or adding toppings like Greek yogurt or almond milk.

Nutritional Information: Calories: 280, Protein: 6g, Carbohydrates: 50g, Fat: 7g, Fiber: 6g, Cholesterol: 0mg, Sodium: 5mg

Vegan Breakfast Tacos with Tofu Scramble

Ingredients

- 1 block (14 oz) firm tofu, drained and crumbled
- 1 tbsp olive oil
- 1/2 tsp turmeric powder
- 1/2 tsp black salt
- 1 small red onion, diced
- 1 red bell pepper, diced
- 1 cup black beans, cooked and drained
- 4 cloves garlic, minced
- 1 tsp cumin powder
- 1/2 tsp chili powder
- Salt and pepper to taste
- 8 small corn tortillas
- Avocado slices, salsa, fresh cilantro (optional toppings)

Prep Time: 15 min

Cook Time: 10 min

Serves: 4

Directions

1. Heat olive oil in a large skillet over medium heat. Add the onion, bell pepper, and garlic. Sauté until the onion becomes translucent, about 5 minutes.

2. Stir in the crumbled tofu, turmeric, black salt, cumin, chili powder, salt, and pepper. Cook for about 10 minutes, stirring occasionally, until the tofu is golden and the spices are fragrant.

3. Warm the tortillas in a dry skillet until they are soft and pliable.

4. Spoon the tofu scramble into each tortilla and add black beans evenly among the tacos.

5. Serve the tacos with optional toppings such as avocado, salsa, and fresh cilantro.

Nutritional Information: Calories: 350, Protein: 18g, Carbohydrates: 45g, Fat: 12g, Fiber: 9g, Cholesterol: 0mg, Sodium: 300mg

Savory Breakfast Muffins

Ingredients

- 2 cups almond flour
- 1 tsp baking powder
- 1/2 tsp salt
- 1/4 tsp black pepper
- 3 large eggs
- 1/4 cup olive oil
- 1/2 cup unsweetened almond milk
- 1 cup chopped spinach
- 1/2 cup diced red bell pepper
- 1/2 cup crumbled feta cheese

Prep Time: 15 min

Cook Time: 25 min

Serves: 6

Directions

1. Preheat the oven to 350°F (175°C). Line a muffin tin with paper liners or grease with a little olive oil.

2. In a large bowl, whisk together the almond flour, baking powder, salt, and pepper.

3. In another bowl, beat the eggs, olive oil, and almond milk together. Add this mixture to the dry ingredients and stir until just combined.

4. Fold in the spinach, red bell pepper, and feta cheese.

5. Divide the batter evenly among the prepared muffin cups, filling each about 3/4 full.

6. Bake in the preheated oven for 25 minutes, or until the tops are golden and a toothpick inserted into the center of a muffin comes out clean.

Nutritional Information: Calories: 320, Protein: 12g, Carbohydrates: 10g, Fat: 27g, Fiber: 4g, Cholesterol: 95mg, Sodium: 370mg

Pumpkin Spice Muffins

Ingredients

- 1 1/2 cups almond flour
- 1/2 cup coconut flour
- 1 tsp baking soda
- 1/4 tsp sea salt
- 2 tsp cinnamon powder
- 1/2 tsp nutmeg powder
- 1/4 tsp clove powder
- 3 large eggs
- 1 cup pumpkin puree (not pumpkin pie filling)
- 1/3 cup unsweetened almond milk
- 1/4 cup melted coconut oil (or avocado oil)
- 1/2 cup maple syrup
- 1 tsp vanilla extract

 Prep Time: 15 min

 Cook Time: 25 min

 Serves: 6

Directions

1. Preheat your oven to 350°F (175°C) and line a muffin tin with paper liners or grease with coconut oil.

2. In a large bowl, whisk together almond flour, coconut flour, baking soda, salt, cinnamon, nutmeg, and cloves.

3. In another bowl, mix together the eggs, pumpkin puree, almond milk, melted coconut oil (or avocado oil), maple syrup, and vanilla extract.

4. Pour the wet ingredients into the dry ingredients and stir until just combined.

5. Divide the batter evenly among the muffin cups, filling each about 3/4 full.

6. Bake in the preheated oven for 25 minutes, or until a toothpick inserted into the center of a muffin comes out clean.

Nutritional Information: Calories: 315, Protein: 9g, Carbohydrates: 28g, Fat: 20g, Fiber: 6g, Cholesterol: 93mg, Sodium: 260mg

Sweet Potato Toast with Blueberries

Ingredients

- 2 large sweet potatoes, sliced lengthwise into 1/4-inch-thick slices
- 1 cup coconut yogurt
- 1/2 cup fresh blueberries
- 2 tbsp chia seeds
- Honey or maple syrup for drizzling (optional)

 Prep Time: 10 min

 Cook Time: 15 min

 Serves: 4

Directions

1. Preheat your toaster or oven to 400°F (200°C). If using an oven, line a baking sheet with parchment paper.

2. Place sweet potato slices in a single layer in the toaster or on the prepared baking sheet. Toast or bake until tender and edges are slightly crispy, about 15 minutes in the oven or several toaster cycles.

3. Spread coconut yogurt evenly over each slice of sweet potato toast.

4. Sprinkle with fresh blueberries and chia seeds.

5. Optional: Drizzle with honey or maple syrup for added sweetness.

Nutritional Information: Calories: 180, Protein: 4g, Carbohydrates: 33g, Fat: 4g, Fiber: 6g, Cholesterol: 0mg, Sodium: 55mg

Goat Cheese Spinach Omelet

Ingredients

- 4 large eggs
- 2 tbsp milk
- 1/4 cup pumpkin seeds, toasted
- 1/4 cup hemp seeds
- 1/2 cup fresh spinach, roughly chopped
- 1/4 cup goat cheese, crumbled
- Salt and pepper to taste
- 1 tbsp olive oil

 Prep Time: 10 min

 Cook Time: 8 min

 Serves: 2

Directions

1. In a medium bowl, whisk together eggs, milk, salt, and pepper until well combined.

2. Heat olive oil in a non-stick skillet over medium heat. Add spinach and sauté until just wilted, about 1-2 minutes.

3. Pour the egg mixture over the spinach. Sprinkle toasted pumpkin seeds and hemp seeds evenly over the top.

4. When the edges start to set, sprinkle crumbled goat cheese over the omelet. Cook for another 3-4 minutes, or until the eggs are set and the bottom is golden brown.

5. Carefully fold the omelet in half and slide onto a plate. Serve immediately.

Nutritional Information: Calories: 450, Protein: 30g, Carbohydrates: 5g, Fat: 34g, Fiber: 2g, Cholesterol: 370mg, Sodium: 320mg

Tuna Salad Stuffed Avocados

Ingredients

- 2 large ripe avocados
- 1 can (5 oz) tuna in water, drained
- 1/4 cup red onion, finely chopped
- 1/4 cup celery, finely chopped
- 2 tbsp plain Greek yogurt
- 1 tbsp Dijon mustard
- Juice of 1/2 a lemon
- Salt and pepper to taste
- Chopped fresh parsley or chives for garnish (optional)

 Prep Time: 15 min

 Cook Time: 0 min

 Serves: 4

Directions

1. Cut the avocados in half lengthwise and remove the pits. Scoop out a bit of the flesh from each half to create more space for the filling, and chop the scooped-out flesh.

2. In a mixing bowl, combine the tuna, chopped avocado, red onion, celery, Greek yogurt, Dijon mustard, and lemon juice. Mix well and season with salt and pepper to taste.

3. Spoon the tuna mixture back into the avocado halves, filling each generously.

4. Garnish with chopped parsley or chives if desired, and serve immediately.

Nutritional Information: Calories: 230, Protein: 10g, Carbohydrates: 12g, Fat: 18g, Fiber: 7g, Cholesterol: 20mg, Sodium: 220mg

Chickpea Pancakes with Salsa

Prep Time: 15 min   Cook Time: 10 min   Serves: 4

Ingredients

For Chickpea Pancakes:
- 1 cup chickpea flour
- 1 cup water
- 1 tsp cumin powder
- 1/2 tsp turmeric powder
- 1/2 tsp baking powder
- 1/4 tsp salt
- 1/4 tsp black pepper
- 1/4 cup chopped fresh cilantro
- 2 tbsp olive oil

For Avocado Salsa:
- 2 ripe avocados, diced
- 1 small red onion, finely chopped
- 1 medium tomato, diced
- 1 jalapeño, finely chopped (optional)
- 1/4 cup chopped fresh cilantro
- Juice of 1 lime
- Salt and pepper

Directions

1. In a mixing bowl, whisk together chickpea flour, water, cumin powder, turmeric powder, baking powder, salt, and black pepper until smooth. Stir in the chopped cilantro.

2. Heat a non-stick skillet over medium heat and add a bit of olive oil. Pour a ladleful of the batter into the skillet, spreading it out to form a thin pancake. Cook for 2-3 minutes on each side until golden brown. Repeat with the remaining batter.

3. In a separate bowl, combine diced avocados, red onion, tomato, jalapeño (If using), cilantro, lime juice, salt, and pepper. Mix gently to make the salsa.

4. Serve the chickpea pancakes warm, topped with generous spoonfuls of avocado salsa.

Nutritional Information: Calories: 350, Protein: 8g, Carbohydrates: 28g, Fat: 24g, Fiber: 10g, Cholesterol: 0mg, Sodium: 250mg

Fire-Roasted Tomatoe Veggie Skillet

Prep Time: 10 min   Cook Time: 25 min   Serves: 4

Ingredients

- 1 large onion, finely chopped
- 1 red bell pepper, diced
- 1 yellow bell pepper, diced
- 3 cloves garlic, minced
- 1 tsp cumin powder
- 1 tsp smoked paprika
- 1/2 tsp chili powder
- 1/2 tsp coriander powder
- 1 can (28 oz) fire-roasted crushed tomatoes
- Crumbled feta cheese
- 2 tbsp extra virgin olive oil
- 1 tsp salt
- 1/2 tsp freshly ground black pepper
- 1/4 cup chopped fresh cilantro
- 4 large eggs
- Fresh parsley, chopped
- 4 gluten-free pita breads
- 1 avocado, sliced

Directions

1. Heat olive oil in a large skillet over medium heat. Add the onion and both bell peppers, and cook until they are soft and starting to caramelize, about 7 minutes. Add garlic, cumin, smoked paprika, chili powder, and coriander, and cook for 1-2 minutes until fragrant.

2. Pour in the crushed tomatoes, salt, and black pepper. Stir in the chopped cilantro. Simmer for 10-15 minutes, allowing the flavors to meld and the sauce to thicken slightly. If the sauce becomes too thick, add a splash of water.

3. Make four small wells in the sauce and carefully crack an egg into each well. Cover the skillet and cook for 5-7 minutes, until the eggs are set to your desired doneness (soft, medium, or hard).

4. While the eggs are cooking, warm pita breads in a toaster or oven, slice the avocado and crumble the feta cheese over eggs.

5. Garnish with fresh parsley and extra cilantro.

Nutritional Information: Calories: 340, Protein: 14g, Carbohydrates: 35g, Fat: 18g, Fiber: 7g, Cholesterol: 200mg, Sodium: 680mg

Chapter 4: Salads

Roasted Pumpkin and Pomegranate Salad

Ingredients

- 4 cups diced pumpkin (about 1 small pumpkin)
- 1 tbsp olive oil
- Salt and pepper to taste
- 2 cups arugula
- 1/2 cup pomegranate seeds
- 1/4 cup toasted pine nuts
- 1/4 cup crumbled feta cheese
- 2 tbsp balsamic vinegar
- 1 tbsp honey

 Prep Time: 15 min

 Cook Time: 30 min

 Serves: 4

Directions

1. Preheat the oven to 400°F (200°C). Toss the diced pumpkin with olive oil, salt, and pepper, then spread on a baking sheet. Roast in the oven for about 30 minutes, or until tender and lightly caramelized.

2. In a large salad bowl, combine the arugula, roasted pumpkin, pomegranate seeds, and toasted pine nuts.

3. Drizzle with balsamic vinegar and honey, then toss gently to coat all ingredients.

4. Sprinkle crumbled feta cheese over the top before serving.

Nutritional Information: Calories: 250, Protein: 6g, Carbohydrates: 30g, Fat: 14g, Fiber: 5g, Cholesterol: 11mg, Sodium: 180mg

Crunchy Carrot and Red Cabbage Salad

Ingredients

- 3 cups grated carrots
- 2 cups shredded red cabbage
- 1 can (15 oz) chickpeas, drained and rinsed
- 1/2 cup raisins
- 1/2 cup sliced almonds, toasted
- 1/4 cup chopped fresh parsley
- 1/4 cup olive oil
- 2 tbsp lemon juice
- 1 tbsp honey
- 1 tsp cumin powder
- 1/2 tsp cinnamon powder
- Salt and pepper to taste

 Prep Time: 20 min

 Cook Time: 0 min

 Serves: 4

Directions

1. In a large bowl, combine the grated carrots, shredded red cabbage, chickpeas, raisins, and toasted almonds.

2. In a small bowl, whisk together the olive oil, lemon juice, honey, cumin, and cinnamon. Season with salt and pepper to taste.

3. Pour the dressing over the salad mixture and toss to coat evenly. Sprinkle with chopped parsley before serving.

Nutritional Information: Calories: 320, Protein: 8g, Carbohydrates: 45g, Fat: 14g, Fiber: 9g, Cholesterol: 0mg, Sodium: 300mg

Lentil and Roasted Beet Salad

Ingredients

- 4 medium beets, peeled and diced
- 1 cup dry green lentils
- 4 cups water
- 1/4 cup olive oil
- 2 tbsp balsamic vinegar
- 1 tsp Dijon mustard
- 1 garlic clove, minced
- Salt and pepper to taste
- 1/4 cup chopped fresh parsley
- 1/4 cup crumbled feta cheese (optional)

 Prep Time: 10 min

 Cook Time: 45 min

 Serves: 4

Directions

1. Preheat the oven to 400°F (200°C). Place the diced beets on a baking sheet, drizzle with 1 tablespoon of olive oil, season with salt and pepper, and toss to coat. Roast for about 30 -35 minutes or until tender and slightly caramelized.

2. While the beets are roasting, rinse the lentils and place them in a saucepan with 4 cups of water. Bring to a boil, then reduce the heat and simmer for 20-25 minutes until the lentils are tender but still hold their shape. Drain any excess water.

3. In a small bowl, whisk together the remaining olive oil, balsamic vinegar, Dijon mustard, minced garlic, salt, and pepper to create the dressing.

4. In a large bowl, combine the roasted beets, cooked lentils, and fresh parsley. Pour over the dressing and toss gently to combine. If using, sprinkle with feta cheese before serving.

Nutritional Information: Calories: 290, Protein: 14g, Carbohydrates: 39g, Fat: 9g, Fiber: 12g, Cholesterol: 8mg, Sodium: 200mg

Roasted Sweet Potato Arugula Salad

Ingredients

- 2 large sweet potatoes, peeled and cubed
- 3 tbsp olive oil, divided
- Salt and black pepper, to taste
- 4 cups arugula
- 1/2 cup pecans, toasted
- 1/4 cup dried cranberries
- 2 tbsp maple syrup
- 1 tbsp balsamic vinegar
- 1 tsp Dijon mustard

 Prep Time: 15 min

 Cook Time: 25 min

 Serves: 4

Directions

1. Preheat the oven to 400°F (200°C). Toss the sweet potato cubes with 2 tablespoons of olive oil, salt, and pepper. Spread on a baking sheet and roast for 25 minutes, or until tender and golden.

2. In a small bowl, whisk together the remaining olive oil, maple syrup, balsamic vinegar, and Dijon mustard to create the vinaigrette. Season with salt and pepper to taste.

3. In a large salad bowl, combine the roasted sweet potatoes, arugula, toasted pecans, and dried cranberries.

4. Drizzle the maple vinaigrette over the salad and toss gently to combine.

Nutritional Information: Calories: 340, Protein: 3g, Carbohydrates: 38g, Fat: 21g, Fiber: 6g, Cholesterol: 0mg, Sodium: 150mg

Quinoa and Black Bean Salad

Ingredients

- 1 cup quinoa (uncooked)
- 2 cups water
- 1 can (15 oz) black beans, drained and rinsed
- 1 medium red bell pepper, diced
- 1 medium red onion, finely chopped
- 1 ripe avocado, diced
- 1/2 cup fresh cilantro, chopped
- 2 tbsp lime juice
- 1/4 cup olive oil
- 1 garlic clove, minced
- Salt and pepper to taste

 Prep Time: 15 min

 Cook Time: 20 min

 Serves: 4

Directions

1. Rinse the quinoa under cold water until the water runs clear. In a medium saucepan, combine the quinoa and water and bring to a boil. Reduce heat to low, cover, and simmer for 15 minutes, or until the water is absorbed. Remove from heat and let stand for 5 minutes, then fluff with a fork.

2. In a large bowl, combine the cooked quinoa, black beans, bell pepper, and onion.

3. In a blender or food processor, combine the avocado, cilantro, lime juice, olive oil, and garlic. Blend until smooth. Season with salt and pepper to taste.

4. Pour the dressing over the quinoa mixture and toss to coat evenly.

5. Serve immediately, or chill in the refrigerator for an hour to allow flavors to meld.

Nutritional Information: Calories: 380, Protein: 12g, Carbohydrates: 54g, Fat: 16g, Fiber: 12g, Cholesterol: 0mg, Sodium: 200mg

Broccoli and Blueberry Salad

Ingredients

- 4 cups fresh broccoli florets
- 1 cup fresh blueberries
- 1/4 cup sunflower seeds
- 1/4 cup finely chopped red onion
- 1/2 cup plain Greek yogurt
- 2 tbsp honey
- 2 tbsp apple cider vinegar
- Salt and pepper to taste

 Prep Time: 15 min

 Cook Time: 0 min

 Serves: 4

Directions

1. In a large bowl, combine the broccoli florets, blueberries, sunflower seeds, and red onion.

2. In a small bowl, whisk together the Greek yogurt, honey, and apple cider vinegar until smooth. Season with salt and pepper to taste.

3. Pour the yogurt dressing over the broccoli mixture and toss to coat evenly. Chill in the refrigerator for at least 30 minutes before serving to allow flavors to meld.

Nutritional Information: Calories: 180, Protein: 6g, Carbohydrates: 23g, Fat: 8g, Fiber: 4g, Cholesterol: 3mg, Sodium: 80mg

Spinach Steak Salad

Ingredients

- 1 lb sirloin steak, about 1-inch thick
- 2 tbsp olive oil
- 4 cups fresh spinach
- 1 cup sliced mushrooms
- 1/4 cup red onion, thinly sliced
- 1/4 cup balsamic vinegar
- 1 tbsp Dijon mustard
- 1 tsp honey
- 1/2 cup extra virgin olive oil
- Salt and pepper to taste
- Crumbled blue cheese or goat cheese (optional)

 Prep Time: 15 min

 Cook Time: 10 min

 Serves: 4

Directions

1. Season the steak with salt and pepper. Heat olive oil in a skillet over medium-high heat. Cook the steak for about 4-5 minutes per side or until desired doneness. Let it rest for 5 minutes before slicing thinly.

2. In the same skillet, add mushrooms and sauté for about 5 minutes until browned and tender. Remove from heat.

3. In a small bowl, whisk together balsamic vinegar, Dijon mustard, honey, and extra virgin olive oil to create the vinaigrette.

4. Toss spinach and red onion in a large bowl, add the cooked mushrooms, and drizzle with the balsamic vinaigrette. Top with sliced steak and optional cheese.

Nutritional Information: Calories: 485, Protein: 32g, Carbohydrates: 8g, Fat: 37g, Fiber: 2g, Cholesterol: 70mg, Sodium: 320mg

Grilled Salmon and Asparagus Salad

Ingredients

- 4 salmon fillets (6 oz each)
- 1 lb asparagus, trimmed
- 2 avocados, sliced
- 2 tbsp olive oil
- Salt and pepper to taste
- 1/4 cup balsamic glaze
- Mixed salad greens or arugula

 Prep Time: 15 min

 Cook Time: 10 min

 Serves: 4

Directions

1. Preheat the grill to medium-high heat. Brush the salmon fillets and asparagus with olive oil, and season with salt and pepper.

2. Grill the salmon for about 4-5 minutes per side or until cooked through. Grill the asparagus alongside, turning occasionally, until tender and charred, about 5-7 minutes.

3. Arrange the mixed greens or arugula on plates. Place grilled asparagus and salmon on top. Add slices of avocado around the salmon.

4. Drizzle each serving with balsamic glaze before serving.

Nutritional Information: Calories: 470, Protein: 35g, Carbohydrates: 14g, Fat: 32g, Fiber: 7g, Cholesterol: 85mg, Sodium: 200mg

Turmeric Roasted Cauliflower Salad

Ingredients

- 1 large head of cauliflower, cut into florets
- 2 tbsp olive oil
- 1 tsp turmeric powder
- Salt and pepper, to taste
- 4 cups mixed greens
- 1/2 cup pomegranate seeds
- 1/4 cup sliced almonds
- 2 tbsp fresh ginger, minced
- 2 tbsp apple cider vinegar
- 1 tbsp honey
- 1 tbsp Dijon mustard
- 1/4 cup extra virgin olive oil

Prep Time: 15 min

Cook Time: 25 min

Serves: 4

Directions

1. Preheat the oven to 400°F (200°C). Toss the cauliflower florets with olive oil, turmeric, salt, and pepper. Spread on a baking sheet and roast for 25 minutes, stirring halfway through, until golden and tender.

2. In a small bowl, whisk together minced ginger, apple cider vinegar, honey, Dijon mustard, and extra virgin olive oil to create the dressing.

3. In a large salad bowl, combine the roasted cauliflower, mixed greens, pomegranate seeds, and sliced almonds.

4. Drizzle the ginger dressing over the salad and toss gently to combine.

Nutritional Information: Calories: 260, Protein: 5g, Carbohydrates: 20g, Fat: 20g, Fiber: 5g, Cholesterol: 0mg, Sodium: 150mg

Roasted Brussels Sprouts Salad

Ingredients

- 1 lb Brussels sprouts, trimmed and halved
- 1/3 cup whole almonds
- 1/4 cup dried cranberries
- 1/4 cup grated Parmesan cheese
- 3 tbsp olive oil
- 2 cloves garlic, minced
- Juice and zest of 1 lemon
- Salt and pepper to taste

Prep Time: 10 min

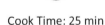

Cook Time: 25 min

Serves: 4

Directions

1. Preheat the oven to 400°F (200°C). Toss the Brussels sprouts with 2 tablespoons of olive oil, salt, and pepper. Spread on a baking sheet and roast for about 20-25 minutes, until caramelized and tender.

2. Meanwhile, in a dry skillet over medium heat, toast the almonds until golden and fragrant, about 5 minutes. Let cool and then roughly chop.

3. In a small bowl, whisk together the remaining tablespoon of olive oil, garlic, lemon juice, and lemon zest to create the dressing.

4. In a large bowl, combine the roasted Brussels sprouts, toasted almonds, dried cranberries, and Parmesan cheese. Drizzle with the garlic-lemon dressing and toss to combine.

Nutritional Information: Calories: 280, Protein: 9g, Carbohydrates: 23g, Fat: 19g, Fiber: 6g, Cholesterol: 7mg, Sodium: 220mg

Lentils Vitality Salad

Ingredients

- 2 cups cooked lentils (preferably green or black lentils)
- 1 large cucumber, diced
- 2 medium tomatoes, diced
- 1/2 cup Kalamata olives, halved
- 1/2 cup crumbled feta cheese
- 1/4 cup red onion, finely chopped
- 3 tbsp red wine vinegar
- 1/4 cup olive oil
- 1 tsp Dijon mustard
- 1 clove garlic, minced
- Salt and pepper to taste
- Fresh parsley, chopped for garnish

 Prep Time: 15 min

 Cook Time: 0 min

 Serves: 4

Directions

1. In a large bowl, combine the cooked lentils, cucumber, tomatoes, olives, feta cheese, and red onion.

2. In a small bowl, whisk together the red wine vinegar, olive oil, Dijon mustard, minced garlic, salt, and pepper to create the vinaigrette.

3. Pour the vinaigrette over the salad and toss gently to coat all the ingredients evenly.

4. Garnish with chopped fresh parsley before serving.

Nutritional Information: Calories: 340, Protein: 14g, Carbohydrates: 30g, Fat: 18g, Fiber: 10g, Cholesterol: 25mg, Sodium: 570mg

Grilled Halloumi and Fig Salad

Ingredients

- 8 oz halloumi cheese, sliced
- 6 fresh figs, quartered
- 4 cups arugula
- 1/2 cup walnuts, toasted
- 2 tbsp balsamic vinegar
- 1 tbsp honey
- 1 tbsp olive oil
- Salt and pepper to taste

 Prep Time: 15 min

Cook Time: 10 min

 Serves: 4

Directions

1. Preheat a grill or grill pan over medium heat. Grill the halloumi slices for about 2-3 minutes on each side until they have nice grill marks and are slightly softened.

2. In a small bowl, whisk together balsamic vinegar, honey, and olive oil. Season with a pinch of salt and pepper to create the dressing.

3. Arrange the arugula on a serving platter or in a salad bowl. Top with grilled halloumi, quartered figs, and toasted walnuts.

4. Drizzle the honey-balsamic dressing over the salad just before serving.

Nutritional Information: Calories: 380, Protein: 19g, Carbohydrates: 27g, Fat: 25g, Fiber: 5g, Cholesterol: 50mg, Sodium: 820mg

Spicy Tofu Cucumber Salad

Ingredients

- 14 oz firm tofu, drained and cubed
- 2 large cucumbers, thinly sliced
- 2 large carrots, julienned or shredded
- 2 tbsp sesame oil
- 3 tbsp soy sauce
- 1 tbsp rice vinegar
- 1 tbsp honey or maple syrup
- 1 tsp chili paste (adjust to taste)
- 1 clove garlic, minced
- 1 tbsp fresh ginger, grated
- 2 tbsp sesame seeds, for garnish
- 2 green onions, thinly sliced, for garnish

Prep Time: 20 min

Cook Time: 10 min

Serves: 4

Directions

1. In a non-stick skillet over medium heat, lightly fry the tofu cubes until golden on all sides, about 5-7 minutes. Remove from heat and set aside to cool.

2. In a large bowl, combine the sliced cucumbers and carrots.

3. In a small bowl, whisk together sesame oil, soy sauce, rice vinegar, honey, chili paste, garlic, and ginger to create the dressing.

4. Pour the dressing over the cucumbers and carrots, and toss to coat well.

5. Add the cooled tofu to the salad and gently mix to combine. Refrigerate for at least 10 minutes to allow flavors to meld.

Nutritional Information: Calories: 230, Protein: 13g, Carbohydrates: 18g, Fat: 12g, Fiber: 3g, Cholesterol: 0mg, Sodium: 870mg

Watermelon Feta Salad

Ingredients

- 4 cups cubed watermelon
- 2 cups arugula
- 1 cup crumbled feta cheese
- 1/4 cup fresh mint leaves, finely chopped
- 1/4 cup balsamic reduction
- 2 tbsp olive oil
- Salt and pepper to taste

Prep Time: 15 min

Cook Time: 0 min

Serves: 4

Directions

1. In a large bowl, combine the cubed watermelon, arugula, and chopped mint.

2. Drizzle with olive oil and gently toss to coat the ingredients evenly.

3. Sprinkle crumbled feta cheese over the top.

4. Drizzle the balsamic reduction over the salad just before serving.

5. Season with a pinch of salt and pepper to taste and serve immediately.

Nutritional Information: Calories: 180, Protein: 5g, Carbohydrates: 18g, Fat: 10g, Fiber: 1g, Cholesterol: 25mg, Sodium: 320mg

Sardine and Roasted Beet Salad

Ingredients

- 4 medium beets, peeled and cubed
- 2 tbsp olive oil
- Salt and pepper to taste
- 4 cups mixed greens
- 2 cans of sardines in olive oil, drained
- 2 oranges, peeled and segmented
- 2 tbsp orange juice
- 1 tbsp Dijon mustard
- 1 tbsp honey
- 3 tbsp extra virgin olive oil

 Prep Time: 15 min

 Cook Time: 30 min

 Serves: 4

Directions

1. Preheat your oven to 400°F (200°C). Toss the beets with olive oil, salt, and pepper, and spread them on a baking sheet. Roast for about 30 minutes, or until tender and slightly caramelized. Allow to cool slightly.

2. In a small bowl, whisk together orange juice, Dijon mustard, honey, and extra virgin olive oil to make the dressing. Season with salt and pepper to taste.

3. In a large bowl, combine the mixed greens, roasted beets, sardines, and orange segments. Drizzle with the orange-mustard dressing and toss gently to combine.

4. Serve the salad immediately, ensuring even distribution of beets, sardines, and orange segments in each serving.

Nutritional Information: Calories: 330, Protein: 15g, Carbohydrates: 23g, Fat: 20g, Fiber: 5g, Cholesterol: 70mg, Sodium: 560mg

Goat Cheese, Beets and Quinoa Salad

Ingredients

- 4 medium beets, peeled and diced
- 1 cup quinoa, rinsed
- 2 cups water
- 4 cups arugula
- 1/2 cup walnuts, toasted and chopped
- 1/2 cup goat cheese, crumbled
- 1/4 cup balsamic reduction
- 2 tbsp olive oil
- Salt and pepper to taste

 Prep Time: 15 min

 Cook Time: 30 min

 Serves: 4

Directions

1. Preheat the oven to 400°F (200°C). Toss the diced beets with 1 tablespoon of olive oil, salt, and pepper. Spread them on a baking sheet and roast for about 25-30 minutes, or until tender and caramelized.

2. While the beets are roasting, combine quinoa and water in a saucepan. Bring to a boil, then reduce heat to low, cover, and simmer for about 15 minutes, or until the quinoa is cooked and water is absorbed. Let cooked quinoa cool.

3. In a large bowl, combine the cooked quinoa, roasted beets, and arugula. Toss with the remaining olive oil and season with salt and pepper.

4. Divide the salad among plates and top with toasted walnuts and crumbled goat cheese. Drizzle with balsamic reduction before serving.

Nutritional Information: Calories: 380, Protein: 13g, Carbohydrates: 40g, Fat: 20g, Fiber: 6g, Cholesterol: 13mg, Sodium: 200mg

Balsamic Chicken and Peach Salad

Ingredients

- 2 large chicken breasts
- Salt and pepper to taste
- 1 tbsp olive oil
- 4 cups mixed greens
- 2 ripe peaches, sliced
- 1/2 cup goat cheese, crumbled
- 1/4 cup balsamic vinegar
- 1 tbsp honey
- 1 tsp Dijon mustard
- 1/3 cup extra virgin olive oil
- Salt and pepper to taste

 Prep Time: 15 min

 Cook Time: 15 min

 Serves: 4

Directions

1. Season the chicken breasts with salt and pepper. Heat olive oil in a skillet over medium heat and cook the chicken until golden and cooked through, about 6-7 minutes per side. Let it rest for a few minutes before slicing.

2. In a small bowl, whisk together balsamic vinegar, honey, Dijon mustard, extra virgin olive oil, salt, and pepper to create the vinaigrette.

3. Arrange the mixed greens on plates and top with sliced chicken, peach slices, and crumbled goat cheese.

4. Drizzle the balsamic vinaigrette over the salad before serving.

Nutritional Information: Calories: 390, Protein: 28g, Carbohydrates: 19g, Fat: 23g, Fiber: 3g, Cholesterol: 75mg, Sodium: 320mg

Roasted Root Vegetable Salad

Ingredients

- 3 medium carrots, peeled and sliced
- 3 medium beets, peeled and cubed
- 2 large sweet potatoes, peeled and cubed
- 3 tbsp olive oil
- Salt and pepper to taste
- 4 cups arugula
- 2 tbsp tahini
- Juice of 1 lemon
- 1 clove garlic, minced
- 2 tbsp warm water
- 1 tbsp honey or maple syrup

 Prep Time: 15 min

 Cook Time: 30 min

 Serves: 4

Directions

1. Preheat your oven to 400°F (200°C). Toss the carrots, beets, and sweet potatoes with olive oil, salt, and pepper. Spread them on a baking sheet and roast in the oven for about 30 minutes, or until tender and caramelized, stirring halfway through cooking.

2. In a small bowl, whisk together the tahini, lemon juice, garlic, warm water, and honey until smooth and creamy.

3. Place the arugula in a large salad bowl and top with the roasted vegetables.

4. Drizzle the lemon-tahini dressing over the salad and toss gently to combine.

Nutritional Information: Calories: 280, Protein: 4g, Carbohydrates: 41g, Fat: 12g, Fiber: 7g, Cholesterol: 0mg, Sodium: 150mg

Asian Tuna Salad

Prep Time: 20 min   Cook Time: 5 min   Serves: 4

Ingredients

- 4 tuna steaks (about 6 oz each)
- 1 tbsp olive oil
- Salt and pepper to taste
- 8 cups mixed greens
- 1 avocado, sliced
- 1 cucumber, sliced
- 4 radishes, thinly sliced
- 2 tbsp sesame seeds

For Ginger Dressing:
- 1/4 cup sesame oil
- 1/4 cup soy sauce
- 2 tbsp rice vinegar
- 1 tbsp honey
- 2 tsp freshly grated ginger
- 1 garlic clove, minced

Directions

1. Heat olive oil in a skillet over medium-high heat. Season the tuna steaks with salt and pepper, and sear for about 2 minutes on each side for medium-rare, or longer depending on your preference. Remove from heat and let rest for a few minutes before slicing thinly.

2. In a small bowl, whisk together the sesame oil, soy sauce, rice vinegar, honey, grated ginger, and minced garlic to create the dressing.

3. Arrange the mixed greens on plates and top with sliced avocado, cucumber, and radishes.

4. Place the sliced tuna on top of the salads and sprinkle with sesame seeds.

5. Drizzle the ginger dressing over each salad just before serving.

Nutritional Information: Calories: 350, Protein: 28g, Carbohydrates: 14g, Fat: 21g, Fiber: 5g, Cholesterol: 45mg, Sodium: 900mg

Beef Salad with Kimchi

Prep Time: 20 min   Cook Time: 10 min   Serves: 4

Ingredients

- 1 lb beef sirloin, thinly sliced
- 4 cups mixed greens
- 1 cup kimchi, chopped
- 2 green onions, thinly sliced
- 1 tbsp sesame seeds
- 2 tbsp soy sauce (or tamari for gluten-free option)
- 1 tbsp honey
- 1 tbsp sesame oil
- 2 cloves garlic, minced
- 1 inch ginger, grated
- 1 tbsp gochujang (Korean chili paste)
- 1 tbsp rice vinegar

Directions

1. In a bowl, combine soy sauce, sesame oil, honey, garlic, ginger, and gochujang to make the marinade. Add the beef slices to the marinade, ensuring they are well coated, and let marinate for at least 15 minutes.

2. Heat a grill pan or skillet over medium-high heat. Remove the beef from the marinade and grill for about 2-3 minutes per side, or until cooked to your liking.

3. In a large bowl, toss the mixed greens with the kimchi, green onions, and grilled beef.

4. For the dressing, whisk together the remaining marinade with rice vinegar. Drizzle over the salad and toss gently to combine.

5. Garnish with sesame seeds before serving.

Nutritional Information: Calories: 250, Protein: 26g, Carbohydrates: 9g, Fat: 12g, Fiber: 2g, Cholesterol: 60mg, Sodium: 690mg

Apple and Fennel Salad

Prep Time: 15 min

Cook Time: 0 min

Serves: 4

Ingredients

- 2 large apples (preferably Granny Smith or Honeycrisp), cored and thinly sliced
- 1 medium fennel bulb, thinly sliced (reserve fronds for garnish)
- 1/4 cup lemon juice
- 1/4 cup extra-virgin olive oil
- 1 tbsp honey
- 1 tsp Dijon mustard
- Salt and pepper to taste
- 1/4 cup toasted walnuts, roughly chopped
- 1/4 cup crumbled feta cheese (optional)

Directions

1. In a large bowl, combine the apple slices and fennel slices.

2. In a small bowl, whisk together the lemon juice, olive oil, honey, Dijon mustard, salt, and pepper until well combined.

3. Pour the dressing over the apple and fennel mixture, tossing to coat evenly.

4. Sprinkle the toasted walnuts and feta cheese (if using) over the salad. Garnish with reserved fennel fronds.

Nutritional Information: Calories: 230, Protein: 3g, Carbohydrates: 24g, Fat: 14g, Fiber: 5g, Cholesterol: 0mg, Sodium: 200mg

Kale Caesar Salad with Grilled Shrimp

Prep Time: 15 min

Cook Time: 30 min

Serves: 4

Ingredients

- 1 pound shrimp, peeled and deveined
- 1 tbsp olive oil
- Salt and black pepper to taste
- 4 cups chopped kale, stems removed
- 1/2 cup shaved Parmesan cheese
- 1 ripe avocado
- 1 clove garlic, minced
- Juice of 1 lemon
- 1/4 cup Greek yogurt
- 2 tbsp water (or as needed for consistency)

Directions

1. Preheat the grill to medium-high heat. Toss the shrimp with olive oil, salt, and pepper. Grill the shrimp for about 2-3 minutes on each side or until cooked through and slightly charred.

2. In a blender, combine the avocado, garlic, lemon juice, Greek yogurt, and a pinch of salt. Blend until smooth, adding water as needed to achieve a creamy dressing consistency.

3. In a large bowl, massage the chopped kale, add the avocado dressing until well coated. Then, add the grilled shrimp and shaved Parmesan cheese to the kale and toss gently to combine.

4. Serve the salad immediately, optionally topped with croutons for added crunch.

Nutritional Information: Calories: 280, Protein: 28g, Carbohydrates: 12g, Fat: 15g, Fiber: 4g, Cholesterol: 180mg, Sodium: 400mg

Chapter 5: Soups & Stews

Split Pea Soup with Turkey Sausage

Ingredients

- 1 cup dried split peas, rinsed
- 6 cups low-sodium chicken broth
- 1/2 pound turkey sausage, sliced into rounds
- 2 carrots, peeled and diced
- 1 onion, chopped
- 2 celery stalks, diced
- 2 garlic cloves, minced
- 1 tsp dried thyme
- 1/2 tsp black pepper
- 1 bay leaf
- 1 tbsp olive oil
- Salt to taste

 Prep Time: 20 min

 Cook Time: 1 hour

Serves: 4

Directions

1. In a large pot, heat the olive oil over medium heat. Add the turkey sausage and cook until browned, about 5 minutes. Remove the sausage and set aside.

2. In the same pot, add the onions, carrots, celery, and garlic. Cook, stirring occasionally, until the vegetables are softened, about 5 minutes.

3. Add the split peas, chicken broth, thyme, black pepper, and bay leaf to the pot. Bring to a boil, then reduce heat to low and simmer for 45 minutes, or until the split peas are tender.

4. Return the sausage to the pot and cook for an additional 10 minutes. Remove the bay leaf before serving. Adjust seasoning with salt if needed.

5. Serve hot.

Nutritional Information: Calories: 345, Protein: 24g, Carbohydrates: 42g, Fat: 9g, Fiber: 16g, Cholesterol: 30mg, Sodium: 680mg

Chickpea and Spinach Stew

Ingredients

- 2 tbsp olive oil
- 1 large onion, chopped
- 2 garlic cloves, minced
- 1/2 tsp turmeric powder
- 1 tsp cumin powder
- 1/2 tsp chili powder
- 1 can (14 oz) diced tomatoes
- 1 can (14 oz) chickpeas, drained and rinsed
- 4 cups vegetable broth
- 4 cups fresh spinach leaves
- Salt and pepper, to taste
- 1 tsp lemon juice

 Prep Time: 15 min

 Cook Time: 30 min

 Serves: 4

Directions

1. Heat the olive oil in a large pot over medium heat. Add the chopped onion and minced garlic, sautéing until the onion is translucent, about 5 minutes.

2. Stir in the turmeric, cumin, and chili powder, cooking for another minute until fragrant.

3. Add the diced tomatoes, chickpeas, and vegetable broth. Bring the mixture to a boil, then reduce the heat and simmer for 20 minutes.

4. Stir in the fresh spinach leaves and continue to simmer until the spinach is wilted, about 5 minutes. Season with salt and pepper, and finish by stirring in the lemon juice. Serve hot.

Nutritional Information: Calories: 210, Protein: 9g, Carbohydrates: 33g, Fat: 5g, Fiber: 9g, Cholesterol: 0mg, Sodium: 300mg

Creamy Cauliflower and Roasted Garlic Soup

 Prep Time: 15 min   Cook Time: 35 min   Serves: 4

Ingredients

- 1 large head of cauliflower, cut into florets
- 1 whole head of garlic, top sliced off to expose cloves
- 2 tbsp olive oil
- 1 medium onion, diced
- 3 cups vegetable broth (low sodium)
- 1 cup light coconut milk
- 1/2 tsp turmeric powder
- Salt and pepper to taste
- Fresh thyme or parsley for garnish (optional)

Directions

1. Preheat the oven to 400°F (200°C). Place cauliflower florets on a baking sheet, drizzle with 1 tablespoon of olive oil, and season with salt and pepper. Wrap the garlic head in foil with a drizzle of olive oil and place it on the baking sheet. Roast in the oven for about 25 minutes or until the cauliflower is golden and tender.

2. Heat the remaining tablespoon of olive oil in a large pot over medium heat. Add diced onion and cook until translucent, about 5 minutes.

3. Add roasted cauliflower, squeezed-out roasted garlic (discard the skins), and turmeric to the pot. Stir to combine.

4. Pour in vegetable broth and bring to a boil. Reduce heat and simmer for 10 minutes.

5. Use an immersion blender to puree the soup until smooth. Stir in coconut milk and adjust seasoning with salt and pepper. Heat through.

6. Serve hot, garnished with fresh thyme or parsley if desired.

Nutritional Information: Calories: 230, Protein: 5g, Carbohydrates: 24g, Fat: 14g, Fiber: 6g, Cholesterol: 0mg, Sodium: 300mg

Lentil and Veggie Healing Stew

 Prep Time: 15 min   Cook Time: 45 min   Serves: 4

Ingredients

- 1 tbsp olive oil
- 1 large onion, diced
- 2 cloves garlic, minced
- 2 carrots, peeled and diced
- 1 red bell pepper, diced
- 1 tsp cumin powder
- 1 tsp coriander powder
- 1/2 tsp turmeric powder
- 4 cups vegetable broth
- 1/4 tsp cayenne pepper (optional, adjust to taste)
- 1 cup dried lentils, rinsed
- 1 (14.5 oz) can diced tomatoes, with their juice
- Salt and black pepper, to taste
- 2 tbsp chopped fresh cilantro, for garnish

Directions

1. Heat the olive oil in a large pot over medium heat. Add the onion and garlic, and sauté until the onions become translucent, about 5 minutes.

2. Add the carrots and red bell pepper to the pot, cooking for another 5 minutes until the vegetables start to soften.

3. Stir in the cumin, coriander, turmeric, and cayenne pepper; cook for 1 minute until fragrant.

4. Add the lentils, diced tomatoes with their juice, and vegetable broth. Bring the mixture to a boil, then reduce the heat to low and simmer, covered, for about 35 minutes, or until the lentils are tender.

5. Season with salt and black pepper to taste. Serve hot, garnished with chopped cilantro.

Nutritional Information: Calories: 310, Protein: 18g, Carbohydrates: 45g, Fat: 5g, Fiber: 18g, Cholesterol: 0mg, Sodium: 300mg

Detoxifying Chicken Soup

Prep Time: 20 min   Cook Time: 40 min   Serves: 4

Ingredients

- 2 tbsp olive oil
- 1 medium onion, chopped
- 3 garlic cloves, minced
- 2 tbsp fresh ginger, minced
- 1/2 tsp turmeric powder
- 1 tsp cumin powder
- 1/2 tsp black pepper
- 4 cups low-sodium chicken broth
- 2 large carrots, sliced
- 2 celery stalks, sliced
- 1 pound chicken breast, skinless and boneless, cut into bite-sized pieces
- 1 cup coconut milk
- Juice of 1 lemon
- Salt to taste
- Fresh cilantro, chopped (for garnish)

Directions

1. In a large pot, heat olive oil over medium heat. Add the onion, garlic, and ginger, sautéing until the onion becomes translucent, about 5 minutes.
2. Stir in the turmeric, cumin, and black pepper, cooking for another minute until fragrant.
3. Add the chicken broth, carrots, and celery. Bring to a boil, then reduce the heat and simmer for 20 minutes.
4. Add the chicken pieces to the pot and continue to simmer until the chicken is fully cooked, about 15 minutes.
5. Stir in the coconut milk and lemon juice, and heat through. Adjust the seasoning with salt.
6. Serve hot, garnished with fresh cilantro.

Nutritional Information: Calories: 310, Protein: 25g, Carbohydrates: 14g, Fat: 17g, Fiber: 3g, Cholesterol: 55mg, Sodium: 400mg

Rainbow Vegetarian Chili

Prep Time: 15 min   Cook Time: 45 min   Serves: 4

Ingredients

- 2 tbsp olive oil
- 1 large onion, chopped
- 2 cloves garlic, minced
- 1 bell pepper, diced
- 2 carrots, peeled and diced
- 2 stalks celery, diced
- 1 zucchini, diced
- 1 sweet potato, peeled and cubed
- 1 can (15 oz) black beans, drained and rinsed
- 1 can (15 oz) kidney beans, drained and rinsed
- 1 can (28 oz) diced tomatoes
- 2 tbsp tomato paste
- 1 tbsp chili powder
- 2 tsp cumin
- 1 tsp smoked paprika
- 1/2 tsp turmeric powder
- Salt and black pepper to taste
- 2 cups vegetable broth
- Chopped cilantro, diced avocado, lime wedges (optional toppings)

Directions

1. In a large pot, heat the olive oil over medium heat. Add the onion and garlic, sautéing until the onion becomes translucent, about 5 minutes.
2. Add the bell pepper, carrots, celery, zucchini, and sweet potato to the pot. Cook for another 5-7 minutes until the vegetables start to soften.
3. Stir in black beans, kidney beans, diced tomatoes, tomato paste, chili powder, cumin, smoked paprika, turmeric, salt, and black pepper. Mix well to combine all the ingredients.
4. Pour in the vegetable broth and bring the chili to a boil. Reduce the heat to low and let it simmer, covered, for about 30 minutes, or until the sweet potatoes are tender and the chili has thickened.
5. Serve hot, with optional toppings like chopped cilantro, diced avocado, and lime wedges if desired.

Nutritional Information: Calories: 340, Protein: 18g, Carbohydrates: 60g, Fat: 5g, Fiber: 20g, Cholesterol: 0mg, Sodium: 500mg

Chicken and White Bean Stew

Prep Time: 15 min   Cook Time: 45 min   Serves: 4

Ingredients

- 2 tbsp olive oil
- 2 chicken breasts, boneless and skinless, cubed
- 1 large onion, chopped
- 2 garlic cloves, minced
- 1 red bell pepper, diced
- 2 carrots, sliced
- 1/2 tsp turmeric powder

- 1 tsp dried thyme
- 1/2 tsp black pepper
- 4 cups low-sodium chicken broth
- 2 cans (15 oz each) white beans, drained and rinsed
- 2 cups baby spinach
- Salt to taste

Directions

1. Heat olive oil in a large pot over medium heat. Add the cubed chicken and cook until lightly browned, about 5-7 minutes. Remove the chicken and set aside.

2. In the same pot, add the onion, garlic, bell pepper, and carrots. Cook until the vegetables are tender, about 8-10 minutes.

3. Stir in the turmeric, thyme, and black pepper, cooking for an additional minute until fragrant.

4. Return the chicken to the pot and add the chicken broth and white beans. Bring to a boil, then reduce heat and simmer for 25 minutes.

5. Add the spinach and cook until wilted, about 2-3 minutes. Season with salt to taste.

Nutritional Information: Calories: 450, Protein: 36g, Carbohydrates: 54g, Fat: 12g, Fiber: 15g, Cholesterol: 65mg, Sodium: 450mg

Creamy Coconut Curry Soup

Prep Time: 15 min   Cook Time: 25 min   Serves: 4

Ingredients

- 1 tbsp coconut oil
- 1 small onion, finely chopped
- 2 cloves garlic, minced
- 1 tbsp fresh ginger, grated
- 1 red bell pepper, thinly sliced
- 1 small zucchini, sliced into half-moons
- 1 carrot, peeled and sliced into thin rounds
- 1 tbsp Thai red curry paste

- 400 ml (13.5 oz) canned coconut milk
- 3 cups vegetable broth
- 1 cup chopped kale
- 1 tbsp soy sauce (or tamari for gluten-free)
- 1 tbsp lime juice
- Fresh cilantro, for garnish
- 1 tbsp maple syrup to taste (optional)

Directions

1. Heat the coconut oil in a large pot over medium heat. Add the onion, garlic, and ginger, and sauté for about 5 minutes until the onion is translucent.

2. Stir in the red bell pepper, zucchini, and carrot. Cook for another 5 minutes, just until the vegetables start to soften.

3. Add the Thai red curry paste and stir for about 1 minute until the vegetables are well coated and the paste is fragrant.

4. Pour in the coconut milk and vegetable broth, and bring the mixture to a simmer. Cook for about 15 minutes, or until the vegetables are tender.

5. Stir in the chopped kale and continue to simmer for another 5 minutes. Finish the soup by adding the soy sauce and lime juice. Adjust seasoning with maple syrup or sugar if desired.

6. Serve hot, garnished with fresh cilantro.

Nutritional Information: Calories: 250, Protein: 5g, Carbohydrates: 20g, Fat: 15g, Fiber: 6g, Cholesterol: 0mg, Sodium: 700mg

Salmon Chowder with Kale and Sweet Potatoes

Prep Time: 20 min   Cook Time: 30 min   Serves: 4

Ingredients

- 2 tbsp olive oil
- 1 medium onion, chopped
- 2 cloves garlic, minced
- 1 large sweet potato, peeled and cubed
- 4 cups low-sodium chicken or vegetable broth
- 1 tsp dried thyme
- 1/2 tsp ground black pepper
- 1/2 tsp paprika
- 1 bay leaf
- 1 bunch kale, stems removed and leaves chopped
- 1 pound salmon fillet, skin removed and cut into chunks
- 1 cup light cream or coconut milk for a dairy-free option
- Salt to taste

Directions

1. In a large pot, heat the olive oil over medium heat. Add the onion and garlic, and sauté until the onions are translucent, about 5 minutes.

2. Add the sweet potato, broth, thyme, black pepper, paprika, and bay leaf. Bring to a boil, then reduce heat and simmer until the sweet potatoes are tender, about 15 minutes.

3. Stir in the kale and salmon, and continue to simmer until the salmon is cooked through, about 10 minutes.

4. Remove the bay leaf, and stir in the cream or coconut milk. Heat through, adjust salt to taste, and serve hot.

Nutritional Information: Calories: 395, Protein: 25g, Carbohydrates: 28g, Fat: 18g, Fiber: 5g, Cholesterol: 55mg, Sodium: 220mg

Hearty Gluten-free Minestrone

Prep Time: 15 min   Cook Time: 40 min   Serves: 4

Ingredients

- 1 tbsp olive oil
- 1 medium onion, chopped
- 2 cloves garlic, minced
- 1 large carrot, diced
- 1 stalk celery, diced
- 1 small zucchini, diced
- 1/2 cup quinoa, rinsed
- 1 can (14.5 oz) diced tomatoes, with juice
- 4 cups low-sodium vegetable broth
- 1 tsp dried basil
- 1 tsp dried oregano
- 1/2 tsp salt
- 1/4 tsp black pepper
- 1 can (15 oz) cannellini beans, drained and rinsed
- 2 cups chopped kale
- 2 tbsp chopped fresh parsley

Directions

1. Heat the olive oil in a large pot over medium heat. Add the onion and garlic, sautéing until the onion is translucent, about 5 minutes.

2. Add the carrot, celery, and zucchini to the pot and cook for another 5 minutes, until slightly softened.

3. Stir in the quinoa, diced tomatoes, vegetable broth, basil, oregano, salt, and pepper. Bring to a boil, then reduce heat and simmer for 20 minutes.

4. Add the cannellini beans and kale to the pot. Continue to simmer for another 15 minutes, or until the quinoa and vegetables are tender.

5. Remove from heat and stir in the fresh parsley before serving.

Nutritional Information: Calories: 280, Protein: 12g, Carbohydrates: 45g, Fat: 5g, Fiber: 10g, Cholesterol: 0mg, Sodium: 430mg

Healing Tomato and Sardine Stew

Prep Time: 15 min   Cook Time: 30 min   Serves: 4

Ingredients

- 2 cans of sardines in olive oil (about 8.5 oz)
- 1 large onion, finely chopped
- 2 cloves garlic, minced
- 1 red bell pepper, diced
- 1 can (14.5 oz) of diced tomatoes
- 2 tbsp tomato paste
- 1 cup vegetable broth
- 1 tsp smoked paprika
- 1/2 tsp crushed red pepper flakes (optional)
- 1 tbsp chopped fresh parsley
- 1 tbsp chopped fresh basil
- Salt and black pepper to taste
- 2 tbsp olive oil

Directions

1. In a large pot, heat the olive oil over medium heat. Add the onion and garlic, and sauté until the onion becomes translucent, about 5 minutes.

2. Stir in the red bell pepper and cook for another 5 minutes until it starts to soften.

3. Add the diced tomatoes, tomato paste, vegetable broth, smoked paprika, and red pepper flakes. Bring to a simmer and cook for 15 minutes.

4. Gently add the sardines to the pot, trying not to break them too much. Simmer for another 10 minutes.

5. Remove from heat and stir in the chopped parsley and basil. Season with salt and black pepper to taste. Let the stew sit for a couple of minutes before serving to allow flavors to meld.

6. Serve with toasted gluten-free bread.

Nutritional Information: Calories: 295, Protein: 23g, Carbohydrates: 15g, Fat: 17g, Fiber: 4g, Cholesterol: 70mg, Sodium: 890mg

Immune-Boosting Lamb Stew

Prep Time: 20 min   Cook Time: 2 hours   Serves: 4

Ingredients

- 1 lb lamb shoulder, cut into cubes
- 2 tbsp olive oil
- 1 large onion, chopped
- 3 cloves garlic, minced
- 1/2 tsp turmeric powder
- 1/2 tsp cinnamon powder
- 1/2 tsp ground ginger
- 1/2 tsp black pepper
- 1 quart low-sodium vegetable broth
- 1 can (14.5 oz) diced tomatoes
- 1 can (15 oz) chickpeas, drained and rinsed
- 3 carrots, chopped
- 1 cup chopped celery
- 1/2 cup chopped dried apricots
- 1/4 cup chopped fresh parsley
- 1/4 cup chopped fresh cilantro
- Salt to taste

Directions

1. Heat the olive oil in a large pot over medium heat. Add the lamb cubes and brown on all sides, about 5-7 minutes. Remove lamb and set aside.

2. In the same pot, add onion and garlic, cooking until the onions are translucent, about 5 minutes. Stir in turmeric, cinnamon, ginger, and black pepper, and cook for another 2 minutes.

3. Return the lamb to the pot along with beef broth and diced tomatoes. Bring to a boil, then reduce heat and simmer covered for 1 hour.

4. Add carrots, celery, and dried apricots to the pot. Continue to simmer for another 30 minutes, or until the vegetables are tender.

5. Stir in the chickpeas and simmer for an additional 5 minutes.

6. Stir in parsley and cilantro just before serving. Adjust seasoning with salt as needed.

Nutritional Information: Calories: 380, Protein: 24g, Carbohydrates: 23g, Fat: 20g, Fiber: 6g, Cholesterol: 75mg, Sodium: 300mg

Beef Stew with Root Vegetables

 Prep Time: 20 min   Cook Time: 2 hours   Serves: 4

Ingredients

- 1 lb beef chuck, cut into 1-inch cubes
- 2 tbsp olive oil
- 2 medium carrots, peeled and diced
- 2 parsnips, peeled and diced
- 1 small sweet potato, peeled and cubed
- 1 onion, chopped
- 2 cloves garlic, minced
- 4 cups beef broth
- 1 cup water
- 2 tsp dried thyme
- 1 bay leaf
- Salt and pepper
- 1/2 cup chopped fresh parsley (for garnish)

Directions

1. In a large pot or Dutch oven, heat the olive oil over medium-high heat. Add the beef and sear until browned on all sides, about 5-7 minutes.

2. Add the onions and garlic to the pot and cook until softened, about 3-4 minutes.

3. Pour in the beef broth and water, then add the carrots, parsnips, sweet potato, thyme, and bay leaf. Bring to a boil, then reduce heat to low and simmer covered for about 2 hours, or until the beef is tender and the vegetables are cooked through.

4. Season with salt and pepper to taste. Remove the bay leaf before serving.

5. Serve hot, garnished with chopped parsley.

Nutritional Information: Calories: 450, Protein: 35g, Carbohydrates: 33g, Fat: 22g, Fiber: 6g, Cholesterol: 85mg, Sodium: 870mg

Spicy Mackerel and Vegetable Soup

 Prep Time: 20 min   Cook Time: 40 min   Serves: 4

Ingredients

- 2 cans (each 6 oz) mackerel, drained and flaked
- 1 tbsp olive oil
- 1 medium onion, chopped
- 2 cloves garlic, minced
- 2 medium carrots, peeled and diced
- 2 stalks celery, diced
- 1 red bell pepper, chopped
- 1 jalapeño, seeded and finely chopped
- 1 can (14.5 oz) diced tomatoes, with juice
- 4 cups low-sodium vegetable broth
- 1 tsp smoked paprika
- 1 tsp cumin powder
- 1/2 tsp black pepper
- 1 tsp salt
- 2 cups chopped kale
- 1/4 cup chopped fresh cilantro

Directions

1. In a large pot, heat the olive oil over medium heat. Add the onion and garlic and sauté until the onion is translucent, about 5 minutes.

2. Add the carrots, celery, red bell pepper, and jalapeño to the pot. Cook for another 5-7 minutes, until the vegetables begin to soften.

3. Stir in the diced tomatoes with their juice, vegetable broth, smoked paprika, cumin, salt, and black pepper. Bring the mixture to a boil, then reduce the heat and simmer for 20 minutes.

4. Add the flaked mackerel and chopped kale to the pot. Continue to simmer for an additional 10 minutes, or until the kale is tender and the flavors are well blended.

5. Remove from heat and stir in the chopped cilantro just before serving.

Nutritional Information: Calories: 295, Protein: 23g, Carbohydrates: 22g, Fat: 12g, Fiber: 5g, Cholesterol: 60mg, Sodium: 680mg

Anti-Inflammatory Chicken Vegetable Soup

Prep Time: 15 min   Cook Time: 30 min   Serves: 4

Ingredients

- 2 tbsp olive oil
- 1 medium onion, chopped
- 2 garlic cloves, minced
- 1 tbsp fresh ginger, minced
- 1 tsp turmeric powder
- 2 medium carrots, sliced
- 2 celery stalks, sliced
- 1 small zucchini, chopped

- 1 cup chopped kale
- 6 cups low-sodium chicken broth
- 2 chicken breasts, skinless and boneless, cut into bite-sized pieces
- Salt and pepper, to taste
- Fresh parsley, chopped, for garnish

Directions

1. Heat the olive oil in a large pot over medium heat. Add the onion, garlic, and ginger, sautéing until the onion becomes translucent, about 5 minutes.

2. Stir in the turmeric, carrots, celery, and zucchini, and cook for another 5 minutes, just until the vegetables start to soften.

3. Add the chicken broth and bring the mixture to a boil. Once boiling, reduce heat to a simmer and add the chicken pieces. Cover and let simmer for 20 minutes, or until the chicken is cooked through.

4. Add the chopped kale and simmer for an additional 5 minutes. Season with salt and pepper to taste.

5. Serve hot, garnished with fresh parsley.

Nutritional Information: Calories: 250, Protein: 28g, Carbohydrates: 18g, Fat: 8g, Fiber: 4g, Cholesterol: 65mg, Sodium: 400mg

Sardine Glass Noodles Broccoli Soup

Prep Time: 15 min   Cook Time: 25 min   Serves: 4

Ingredients

- 2 (4-oz) cans of sardines in olive oil
- 1 head of broccoli, cut into florets
- 2 cups of kale, chopped
- 4 oz glass noodles
- 1 medium onion, diced
- 2 cloves garlic, minced
- 1-inch piece of ginger, grated
- 6 cups vegetable or chicken broth

- 1 tbsp soy sauce (or tamari for gluten-free)
- 1 tbsp olive oil
- 1 tsp sesame oil
- 1/2 tsp turmeric powder
- 1 tsp black pepper
- 1/2 tsp chili flakes (optional)
- Salt to taste
- Fresh lemon wedges for serving

Directions

1. Heat olive oil in a large pot over medium heat. Add diced onion, minced garlic, and grated ginger, sautéing until fragrant and onions are translucent, about 5 minutes.

2. Add the vegetable or chicken broth, soy sauce, turmeric powder, black pepper, and chili flakes (if using). Bring to a boil, then reduce to a simmer.

3. Add broccoli florets and chopped kale to the pot, cooking until they are tender but still vibrant, about 10 minutes.

4. While the vegetables are cooking, prepare the glass noodles according to package instructions. Drain and set aside.

5. Add the sardines (including the oil from the cans) and cooked glass noodles to the pot, gently stirring to combine. Simmer for another 5 minutes to allow flavors to meld. Drizzle with sesame oil before serving and garnish with fresh lemon wedges.

Nutritional Information: Calories: 320, Protein: 22g, Carbohydrates: 28g, Fat: 15g, Fiber: 5g, Cholesterol: 45mg, Sodium: 720mg

Hearty Barley and Vegetable Soup

 Prep Time: 15 min   Cook Time: 40 min   Serves: 4

Ingredients

- 1 cup pearled barley, rinsed
- 2 tbsp olive oil
- 1 medium onion, diced
- 2 cloves garlic, minced
- 1 carrot, diced
- 1 stalk celery, diced
- 1 zucchini, diced
- 1 red bell pepper, diced
- 1 can (14.5 oz) diced tomatoes, with juice
- 4 cups vegetable broth
- 2 cups water
- 1 tsp dried basil
- 1 tsp dried oregano
- Salt and black pepper to taste
- 1 cup chopped spinach
- 1/4 cup chopped fresh parsley

Directions

1. In a large pot, heat the olive oil over medium heat. Add the onion and garlic, and sauté until the onions become translucent, about 5 minutes.

2. Add the carrot, celery, zucchini, and red bell pepper to the pot. Cook, stirring occasionally, for about 10 minutes, or until the vegetables start to soften.

3. Stir in the diced tomatoes with their juice, vegetable broth, water, barley, basil, and oregano. Bring to a boil. Reduce the heat to low and simmer, covered, for about 25 minutes, or until the barley is tender.

4. Add the chopped spinach and cook for an additional 5 minutes.

5. Season with salt and black pepper to taste. Stir in the fresh parsley just before serving.

Nutritional Information: Calories: 330, Protein: 10g, Carbohydrates: 63g, Fat: 7g, Fiber: 13g, Cholesterol: 0mg, Sodium: 580mg

Chicken Tortilla Less Soup

 Prep Time: 15 min   Cook Time: 30 min   Serves: 4

Ingredients

- 2 tbsp olive oil
- 1 medium onion, chopped
- 2 garlic cloves, minced
- 1 red bell pepper, chopped
- 1 jalapeño, seeded and finely chopped (optional)
- 1 tsp cumin powder
- 1 tsp smoked paprika
- 1/2 tsp coriander powder
- 1/4 tsp cayenne pepper (optional)
- 4 cups low-sodium chicken broth
- 2 cups cooked, shredded chicken breast
- 1 can (14.5 oz) fire-roasted diced tomatoes
- 1 cup frozen corn kernels
- Juice of 1 lime
- Salt and pepper, to taste
- Fresh cilantro, chopped (for garnish)
- Avocado slices (for garnish)

Directions

1. Heat the olive oil in a large pot over medium heat. Add the onion, garlic, red bell pepper, and jalapeño (if using). Sauté until the vegetables are softened, about 5-7 minutes.

2. Stir in the cumin, smoked paprika, coriander, and cayenne pepper, cooking for an additional minute until fragrant.

3. Add the chicken broth, shredded chicken, and diced tomatoes. Bring to a boil, then reduce heat and simmer for 20 minutes.

4. Add the corn and simmer for an additional 5 minutes. Remove from heat and stir in the lime juice. Season with salt and pepper to taste.

5. Serve hot, garnished with chopped cilantro and avocado slices.

Nutritional Information: Calories: 275, Protein: 26g, Carbohydrates: 22g, Fat: 8g, Fiber: 4g, Cholesterol: 58mg, Sodium: 410mg

Slimming Vegetarian Borscht

Prep Time: 20 min   Cook Time: 1.5 hours   Serves: 4

Ingredients

- 2 medium beets, peeled and cubed
- 1 large carrot, peeled and grated
- 1 medium onion, finely chopped
- 2 garlic cloves, minced
- 1/2 head of medium cabbage, shredded
- 1 large potato, peeled and cubed
- 1/2 cup diced tomatoes (canned or fresh)
- 4 cups vegetable broth
- 1 tbsp extra-virgin olive oil
- 1 bay leaf
- 1 tsp dried dill
- Salt and pepper to taste
- Sour cream (optional, for serving)
- Fresh dill, chopped (for garnish)

Directions

1. In a large pot, heat the olive oil over medium heat. Add the onions and garlic, sautéing until the onions become translucent, about 5 minutes.

2. Add the grated carrots, beets, cabbage, and potatoes to the pot. Stir to combine and cook for 10 minutes, stirring occasionally.

3. Pour in the vegetable broth, add diced tomatoes, and bay leaf. Bring the mixture to a boil, then reduce heat to a simmer. Cover and let simmer for about 75 minutes or until all vegetables are tender.

4. Remove the bay leaf, add salt, pepper, and dried dill. Adjust seasoning to taste.

5. Serve hot, garnished with fresh dill and a dollop of sour cream if desired.

Nutritional Information: Calories: 220, Protein: 6g, Carbohydrates: 40g, Fat: 4g, Fiber: 8g, Cholesterol: 0mg, Sodium: 480mg

Savory Salmon and Garden Veggie Stew

Prep Time: 15 min   Cook Time: 45 min   Serves: 4

Ingredients

- 2 tbsp olive oil
- 1 medium onion, chopped
- 2 cloves garlic, minced
- 1 cup dried lentils, rinsed
- 1 large carrot, diced
- 1 red bell pepper, chopped
- 1 zucchini, chopped
- 4 cups vegetable broth
- 1 tsp dried thyme
- 1 tsp dried oregano
- 1/2 tsp black pepper
- 1/2 tsp salt (optional, to taste)
- 1 can (14.5 oz) diced tomatoes
- 4 salmon fillets (about 4 oz each)
- 2 cups baby spinach
- Juice of 1 lemon

Directions

1. In a large pot, heat the olive oil over medium heat. Add the onion and garlic, sautéing until the onions are translucent, about 5 minutes.

2. Add the lentils, carrot, red bell pepper, zucchini, vegetable broth, thyme, oregano, black pepper, and tomatoes. Bring the mixture to a boil, then reduce the heat and simmer, covered, for 30 minutes.

3. Season the salmon fillets with a pinch of salt and black pepper. Place the salmon on top of the lentils, cover, and continue to simmer for 10-15 minutes or until the salmon is cooked through and flakes easily with a fork.

4. Stir in the spinach and cook until wilted, about 2 minutes. Remove from heat and stir in the fresh lemon juice.

5. Serve warm, ensuring each plate receives a salmon fillet and an equal portion of the stew.

Nutritional Information: Calories: 410, Protein: 34g, Carbohydrates: 40g, Fat: 14g, Fiber: 16g, Cholesterol: 55mg, Sodium: 560mg

Chapter 6: Fish & Seafood

Grilled Salmon with Avocado Salsa

Ingredients

- 4 salmon fillets (6 oz each)
- 2 tbsp olive oil
- 1 tsp paprika
- 1 tsp garlic powder
- Salt and pepper to taste
- 2 ripe avocados, diced
- 1 small red onion, finely chopped
- 1 large tomato, diced
- 1/4 cup fresh cilantro, chopped
- Juice of 1 lime
- Salt and pepper to taste

 Prep Time: 15 min

 Cook Time: 10 min

 Serves: 4

Directions

1. Preheat the grill to medium-high heat. Brush the salmon fillets with olive oil and season with paprika, garlic powder, salt, and pepper.

2. Place the salmon fillets on the grill and cook for 4-5 minutes on each side, or until the fish is cooked through and flakes easily with a fork.

3. While the salmon is grilling, prepare the avocado salsa. In a mixing bowl, combine the diced avocado, red onion, tomato, cilantro, lime juice, salt, and pepper. Gently toss to combine.

4. Once the salmon is cooked, remove it from the grill and transfer to serving plates. Top each fillet with a generous spoonful of avocado salsa.

5. Serve immediately, garnished with additional cilantro and lime wedges if desired.

Nutritional Information: Calories: 350, Protein: 30g, Carbohydrates: 10g, Fat: 22g, Fiber: 6g, Cholesterol: 80mg, Sodium: 300mg

Baked Cod with Crispy Garlic Broccoli

Ingredients

- 4 cod fillets (about 6 oz each)
- 1 pound broccoli florets
- 4 cloves garlic, minced
- 2 tbsp olive oil
- 1 tsp lemon zest
- 1 tbsp lemon juice
- Salt and pepper, to taste
- Fresh parsley, for garnish

 Prep Time: 10 min

 Cook Time: 20 min

 Serves: 4

Directions

1. Preheat your oven to 400°F (200°C). Line a baking sheet with parchment paper.

2. Place the cod fillets on the prepared baking sheet. Season with salt, pepper, and half of the minced garlic.

3. In a large bowl, toss the broccoli florets with the remaining minced garlic, olive oil, lemon zest, lemon juice, salt, and pepper until well coated.

4. Spread the broccoli evenly around the cod fillets on the baking sheet.

5. Bake in the preheated oven for 15-20 minutes, or until the cod is cooked through and flakes easily with a fork, and the broccoli is tender but still crisp.

6. Garnish with fresh parsley before serving.

Nutritional Information: Calories: 280, Protein: 30g, Carbohydrates: 15g, Fat: 12g, Fiber: 5g, Cholesterol: 50mg, Sodium: 350mg

Tuna Steaks with Ginger-Lime Sauce

Ingredients

- 4 tuna steaks, about 6 oz each
- 2 tbsp olive oil
- Salt and pepper to taste

For the Ginger-Lime Sauce:

- 2 tbsp soy sauce (use tamari for gluten-free)
- 1 tbsp fresh lime juice
- 1 tbsp grated ginger
- 1 garlic clove, minced
- 1 tbsp honey or maple syrup
- 1 tsp sesame oil
- 1/4 tsp red pepper flakes
- Chopped green onions and sesame seeds for garnish

Prep Time: 10 min

Cook Time: 8 min

Serves: 4

Directions

1. In a small bowl, whisk together the soy sauce, lime juice, grated ginger, minced garlic, honey or maple syrup, sesame oil, and red pepper flakes (if using) to make the Ginger-Lime Sauce. Set aside.

2. Pat the tuna steaks dry with paper towels and season them generously with salt and pepper.

3. Heat the olive oil in a large skillet over medium-high heat until shimmering but not smoking.

4. Carefully place the tuna steaks in the skillet and sear for 2-3 minutes on each side for medium-rare, or until cooked to your desired doneness.

5. Remove the tuna steaks from the skillet and let them rest for a few minutes.

6. Slice and serve the seared tuna steaks drizzled with the Ginger-Lime Sauce and garnished with chopped green onions and sesame seeds.

Nutritional Information: Calories: 285, Protein: 36g, Carbohydrates: 6g, Fat: 12g, Fiber: 0g, Cholesterol: 77mg, Sodium: 582mg

Lemon Garlic Butter Shrimp

Ingredients

- 1 pound large shrimp, peeled and deveined
- 4 cloves garlic, minced
- 2 tbsp olive oil
- 2 tbsp unsalted butter
- Juice of 1 lemon
- 1 tsp lemon zest
- Salt and pepper to taste
- Chopped fresh parsley for garnish

Prep Time: 10 min

Cook Time: 10 min

Serves: 4

Directions

1. In a large bowl, toss the shrimp with minced garlic, olive oil, lemon juice, lemon zest, salt, and pepper until evenly coated. Let it marinate for 5-10 minutes.

2. Heat a skillet over medium-high heat. Add the butter and let it melt.

3. Add the marinated shrimp to the skillet in a single layer, making sure not to overcrowd the pan. Cook for 2-3 minutes on each side until the shrimp turns pink and opaque.

4. Once the shrimp is cooked through, remove from heat and garnish with chopped fresh parsley.

5. Serve immediately, optionally with steamed vegetables or over a bed of quinoa or brown rice.

Nutritional Information: Calories: 220, Protein: 24g, Carbohydrates: 2g, Fat: 13g, Fiber: 0g, Cholesterol: 195mg, Sodium: 290mg

Smoky Chickpeas and Kale Roasted Salmon

Ingredients

- 4 salmon fillets (about 6 oz each)
- 1 can (15 oz) chickpeas, drained and rinsed
- 1 pint cherry tomatoes, halved
- 2 cups kale, chopped
- 1 red onion, thinly sliced
- 2 tbsp olive oil
- 1 tsp smoked paprika
- 1 tsp ground cumin
- 1/2 tsp garlic powder
- Salt and pepper, to taste
- ½ lemon, juiced (plus extra lemon wedges for serving)

 Prep Time: 8 min

 Cook Time: 22 min

 Serves: 4

Directions

1. Preheat the oven to 400°F (200°C) and line a baking sheet with parchment paper. Place salmon fillets on the sheet, drizzle with 1 tablespoon olive oil, and season with salt and pepper. Set aside.

2. In a large bowl, toss the chickpeas, cherry tomatoes, kale, and red onion with the smoked paprika, cumin, garlic powder, salt, pepper, and the remaining olive oil. Make sure everything is well-coated in the spices.

3. Spread the chickpea-kale mixture evenly around the salmon on the baking sheet. Roast for 20-22 minutes, or until the salmon is golden, cooked through, and flakes easily with a fork. The chickpeas should be crispy and the kale lightly charred.

4. Remove from the oven and squeeze lemon juice over the entire dish. Serve the roasted salmon with the smoky chickpea-kale mix and garnish with extra lemon wedges for a zesty kick.

Nutritional Information: Calories: 510, Protein: 47g, Carbohydrates: 29g, Fat: 26g, Fiber: 9g, Cholesterol: 85mg, Sodium: 570mg

Baked Mackerel with Citrus and Olive Oil

Ingredients

- 4 mackerel fillets
- 2 tbsp olive oil
- 2 cloves garlic, minced
- Zest and juice of 1 lemon
- Zest and juice of 1 orange
- 1 tsp dried thyme
- Salt and pepper, to taste
- Fresh parsley, chopped, for garnish

 Prep Time: 10 min

 Cook Time: 15 min

 Serves: 4

Directions

1. Preheat the oven to 400°F (200°C). Line a baking sheet with parchment paper.

2. Place the mackerel fillets on the prepared baking sheet.

3. In a small bowl, whisk together the olive oil, minced garlic, lemon zest and juice, orange zest and juice, dried thyme, salt, and pepper.

4. Pour the citrus and olive oil mixture over the mackerel fillets, making sure they are evenly coated.

5. Bake in the preheated oven for 12-15 minutes, or until the mackerel is cooked through and flakes easily with a fork.

6. Remove from the oven and garnish with fresh chopped parsley before serving.

Nutritional Information: Calories: 290, Protein: 25g, Carbohydrates: 2g, Fat: 20g, Fiber: 1g, Cholesterol: 80mg, Sodium: 220mg

Roasted Sea Bass with Ginger Soy Glaze

Prep Time: 10 min   Cook Time: 15 min   Serves: 4

Ingredients

- 4 sea bass fillets (about 6 oz each)
- 2 tbsp low-sodium soy sauce
- 1 tbsp honey or maple syrup
- 1 tbsp grated fresh ginger
- 2 cloves garlic, minced
- 1 tbsp sesame oil

- 1 tbsp rice vinegar
- 1 tsp ground flaxseeds or rice flour (optional, for thickening)
- Salt and pepper, to taste
- Sesame seeds and chopped green onions for garnish

Directions

1. Preheat the oven to 400°F (200°C). Line a baking sheet with parchment paper or lightly grease it.

2. In a small bowl, whisk together the soy sauce, honey or maple syrup, grated ginger, minced garlic, sesame oil, and rice vinegar. If desired, mix in ground flaxseeds or rice flour to thicken the glaze.

3. Place the sea bass fillets on the prepared baking sheet and season with salt and pepper.

4. Brush the ginger soy glaze generously over the fillets, covering them completely.

5. Roast the sea bass in the preheated oven for 12-15 minutes, or until the fish is cooked through and flakes easily with a fork.

6. Once done, remove the sea bass from the oven and garnish with sesame seeds and chopped green onions.

7. Serve hot with your choice of side dishes.

Nutritional Information: Calories: 285, Protein: 35g, Carbohydrates: 7g, Fat: 12g, Fiber: 1g, Cholesterol: 80mg, Sodium: 460mg

Chili-Lime Cod with Avocado Crema

Prep Time: 10 min   Cook Time: 15 min   Serves: 4

Ingredients

- 4 cod fillets (about 6 oz each)
- 2 tbsp olive oil
- 2 cloves garlic, minced
- 1 tsp chili powder
- 1/2 tsp paprika
- 1/2 tsp cumin powder
- Zest and juice of 1 lime
- Salt and pepper to taste

For Avocado Crema:

- 1 ripe avocado
- 1/4 cup Greek yogurt
- Juice of 1 lime
- Salt and pepper to taste
- Chopped cilantro, lime wedges (optional garnish)

Directions

1. Preheat the oven to 400°F (200°C). Line a baking sheet with parchment paper or lightly grease it with olive oil.

2. In a small bowl, mix together the olive oil, minced garlic, chili powder, paprika, cumin, lime zest, lime juice, salt, and pepper.

3. Place the cod fillets on the prepared baking sheet. Brush each fillet generously with the chili-lime mixture, coating both sides.

4. Bake the cod in the preheated oven for 12-15 minutes, or until the fish is opaque and flakes easily with a fork.

5. While the cod is baking, prepare the avocado crema. In a blender or food processor, combine the avocado, Greek yogurt, lime juice, salt, and pepper. Blend until smooth and creamy.

6. Serve the chili-lime cod hot, topped with a dollop of avocado crema and garnished with chopped cilantro and lime wedges if desired.

Nutritional Information: Calories: 300, Protein: 28g, Carbohydrates: 10g, Fat: 18g, Fiber: 5g, Cholesterol: 60mg, Sodium: 350mg

Halibut Skewers with Green Tomato Salsa

Ingredients

- 1 lb halibut fillets, cut into cubes
- Wooden or metal skewers
- 2 green tomatoes, diced
- 1/4 cup red onion, finely chopped
- 1 jalapeno pepper, seeded and minced
- 1/4 cup fresh cilantro, chopped
- Juice of 1 lime
- 1 tbsp olive oil
- Salt and pepper to taste

 Prep Time: 15 min

 Cook Time: 10 min

 Serves: 4

Directions

1. Preheat your grill to medium-high heat or prepare a grill pan on the stovetop.
2. Thread the halibut cubes onto skewers, leaving a little space between each piece.
3. In a bowl, combine the diced green tomatoes, red onion, jalapeno pepper, cilantro, lime juice, olive oil, salt, and pepper to make the salsa. Mix well.
4. Place the halibut skewers on the grill or grill pan and cook for 3-4 minutes per side, or until the fish is cooked through and flakes easily with a fork.
5. Serve the halibut skewers hot off the grill, topped with the green tomato salsa.

Nutritional Information: Calories: 200, Protein: 25g, Carbohydrates: 6g, Fat: 8g, Fiber: 2g, Cholesterol: 60mg, Sodium: 300mg

Baked Sea Bass with Fennel and Tomato

Ingredients

- 4 medium sea bass fillets
- 2 fennel bulbs, thinly sliced
- 2 tomatoes, sliced
- 2 cloves garlic, minced
- 2 tbsp olive oil
- 1 lemon, sliced
- Salt and pepper to taste
- Fresh parsley for garnish

 Prep Time: 15 min

 Cook Time: 25 min

 Serves: 4

Directions

1. Preheat your oven to 400°F (200°C).
2. Season the sea bass fillets with salt and pepper, then place them in a baking dish.
3. In a bowl, toss together the sliced fennel, sliced tomatoes, minced garlic, and olive oil. Season with salt and pepper.
4. Arrange the fennel and tomato mixture around the sea bass fillets in the baking dish. Place lemon slices on top of each fillet.
5. Bake in the preheated oven for 20-25 minutes, or until the fish is cooked through and flakes easily with a fork.
6. Garnish with fresh parsley before serving.

Nutritional Information: Calories: 280, Protein: 30g, Carbohydrates: 10g, Fat: 14g, Fiber: 4g, Cholesterol: 60mg, Sodium: 350mg

Garlic-Lime Mahi Mahi

Ingredients

- 4 Mahi Mahi fillets (about 6 oz each)
- 3 cloves garlic, minced
- Zest and juice of 2 limes
- 2 tbsp olive oil
- 1 tsp cumin powder
- 1/2 tsp paprika
- Salt and pepper to taste
- Fresh cilantro for garnish (optional)

 Prep Time: 10 min

 Cook Time: 10 min

 Serves: 4

Directions

1. In a small bowl, combine the minced garlic, lime zest, lime juice, olive oil, cumin, paprika, salt, and pepper to make the marinade.

2. Place the Mahi Mahi fillets in a shallow dish or resealable plastic bag and pour the marinade over them. Ensure the fish is evenly coated. Marinate in the refrigerator for at least 30 minutes, or up to 2 hours.

3. Heat a grill or grill pan over medium-high heat. Remove the Mahi Mahi fillets from the marinade and discard any excess marinade.

4. Grill the Mahi Mahi fillets for 4-5 minutes per side, or until they are opaque and easily flake with a fork.

5. Serve hot, with your preferred side and garnished with fresh cilantro if desired.

Nutritional Information: Calories: 230, Protein: 34g, Carbohydrates: 2g, Fat: 10g, Fiber: 0g, Cholesterol: 115mg, Sodium: 280mg

Grilled Swordfish with Roasted Pepper Sauce

Ingredients

- 4 swordfish fillets (about 6 oz each)
- Salt and pepper to taste
- 2 red bell peppers, halved and seeded
- 2 tbsp olive oil
- 2 cloves garlic, minced
- 1 tsp dried oregano
- 1/2 tsp smoked paprika
- Juice of 1 lemon
- Fresh parsley for garnish

 Prep Time: 15 min

Cook Time: 15 min

Serves: 4

Directions

1. Preheat the grill to medium-high heat. Season the swordfish fillets with salt and pepper.

2. Place the red bell pepper halves on the grill, skin side down. Grill for about 8-10 minutes, or until the skin is charred and the peppers are tender. Remove from the grill and let cool slightly.

3. In a blender or food processor, combine the grilled red peppers, olive oil, minced garlic, dried oregano, smoked paprika, and lemon juice. Blend until smooth. Season with salt and pepper to taste.

4. Brush both sides of the swordfish fillets with the roasted pepper sauce.

5. Place the swordfish fillets on the grill and cook for 4-5 minutes per side, or until the fish is cooked through and easily flakes with a fork.

6. Serve the grilled swordfish hot, garnished with fresh parsley, and with any remaining roasted pepper sauce on the side.

Nutritional Information: Calories: 320, Protein: 34g, Carbohydrates: 5g, Fat: 18g, Fiber: 1g, Cholesterol: 80mg, Sodium: 450mg

Baked Sardines with Olives and Herbs

Prep Time: 10 min | Cook Time: 15 min | Serves: 4

Ingredients

- 8 fresh sardines, cleaned and gutted
- 2 tbsp olive oil
- 2 cloves garlic, minced
- 1 lemon, thinly sliced
- 1 tsp dry oregano
- 1 tsp paprika
- 1 tsp dry onion flakes
- 2 tbsp fresh parsley, chopped
- 1/4 cup olives, pitted and sliced
- Salt and pepper to taste

Directions

1. Preheat the oven to 400°F (200°C). Line a baking sheet with parchment paper or lightly grease it.

2. Place the cleaned sardines on the prepared baking sheet. Drizzle with olive oil and sprinkle minced garlic over them.

3. Arrange lemon slices on top of the sardines. Sprinkle with dry oregano, paprika, and dry onion flakes. Scatter sliced olives around the sardines.

4. Season with salt and pepper to taste.

5. Bake in the preheated oven for 12-15 minutes, or until the sardines are cooked through and easily flake with a fork.

6. Once they are ready you can sprinkle with fresh parsley and a squeeze of lemon.

Nutritional Information: Calories: 210, Protein: 18g, Carbohydrates: 2g, Fat: 15g, Fiber: 1g, Cholesterol: 60mg, Sodium: 280mg

Haddock with Tomato Relish

Prep Time: 10 min | Cook Time: 15 min | Serves: 4

Ingredients

- 4 haddock fillets (about 6 oz each)
- 2 tsp paprika
- 1 tsp garlic powder
- 1 tsp onion powder
- 1/2 tsp salt
- 1/4 tsp black pepper
- 2 tbsp olive oil

For Tomato Relish:

- 2 large tomatoes, diced
- 1/4 cup diced red onion
- 2 tbsp chopped fresh parsley
- 1 tbsp balsamic vinegar
- Salt and pepper to taste

Directions

1. Preheat the oven to 400°F (200°C). Line a baking sheet with parchment paper or lightly grease with olive oil.

2. In a small bowl, mix together the paprika, garlic powder, onion powder, salt, and black pepper.

3. Pat the haddock fillets dry with paper towels. Rub both sides of each fillet with the spice mixture.

4. Heat the olive oil in a large skillet over medium-high heat. Once hot, add the haddock fillets and cook for 2-3 minutes on each side until lightly browned.

5. Transfer the browned haddock fillets to the prepared baking sheet. Bake in the preheated oven for 8-10 minutes, or until the fish flakes easily with a fork.

6. For tomato relish in a medium bowl, combine the diced tomatoes, red onion, chopped parsley, and balsamic vinegar. Season with salt and pepper to taste.

7. Serve the paprika-rubbed haddock hot, topped with a generous spoonful of tomato relish.

Nutritional Information: Calories: 250, Protein: 25g, Carbohydrates: 8g, Fat: 12g, Fiber: 2g, Cholesterol: 60mg, Sodium: 480mg

Clams Stir-Fry with Bell Peppers

Ingredients

- 1 pound fresh clams, cleaned and scrubbed
- 2 tbsp olive oil
- 2 bell peppers, sliced
- 2 cups chopped leafy greens (such as Swiss chard or kale)
- 1 cup mushrooms, sliced
- 1 cup sweet peas
- 4 cloves garlic, minced
- 2 tbsp low-sodium soy sauce
- 1 tbsp rice vinegar
- 1 tsp sesame oil
- Salt and pepper to taste
- Red pepper flakes (optional for heat)

 Prep Time: 15 min

 Cook Time: 15 min

 Serves: 4

Directions

1. Heat 1 tablespoon of olive oil in a large skillet or wok over medium-high heat. Add the clams and cook for 3-4 minutes, or until they start to open. Remove the clams from the skillet and set aside, discarding any that do not open.

2. In the same skillet, add the remaining tablespoon of olive oil. Add the bell peppers, leafy greens, mushrooms, sweet peas, and minced garlic. Stir-fry for 5-6 minutes, or until the vegetables are tender-crisp.

3. Return the clams to the skillet with the vegetables. Add the soy sauce, rice vinegar, sesame oil, salt, pepper, and red pepper flakes if using. Stir well to combine and cook for an additional 2-3 minutes, or until everything is heated through.

4. Remove from heat and serve hot.

Nutritional Information: Calories: 280, Protein: 20g, Carbohydrates: 25g, Fat: 10g, Fiber: 8g, Cholesterol: 60mg, Sodium: 480mg

Cajun Shrimp Skillet

Ingredients

- 1 pound large shrimp, peeled and deveined
- 2 tbsp Cajun seasoning
- 2 tbsp olive oil
- 2 cloves garlic, minced
- 1 bell pepper, thinly sliced
- 1 onion, thinly sliced
- 1 zucchini, sliced
- Salt and pepper to taste
- Fresh parsley for garnish

 Prep Time: 10 min

 Cook Time: 10 min

 Serves: 4

Directions

1. In a bowl, toss the shrimp with Cajun seasoning until evenly coated.

2. Heat olive oil in a large skillet over medium-high heat. Add the minced garlic and cook for 1 minute until fragrant.

3. Add the seasoned shrimp to the skillet and cook for 2-3 minutes per side until pink and cooked through. Remove shrimp from the skillet and set aside.

4. In the same skillet, add the sliced bell pepper, onion, and zucchini. Cook for 5-6 minutes, stirring occasionally, until the vegetables are tender.

5. Return the cooked shrimp to the skillet, toss with the vegetables, and cook for an additional minute to heat through. Season with salt and pepper to taste.

6. Garnish with fresh parsley before serving.

Nutritional Information: Calories: 220, Protein: 24g, Carbohydrates: 9g, Fat: 10g, Fiber: 2g, Cholesterol: 180mg, Sodium: 400mg

Salmon Fillets with Walnut Crust

Ingredients

- 4 salmon fillets (about 6 oz each), skin removed
- 1/2 cup walnuts, finely chopped
- 1 tbsp Dijon mustard
- 1 tbsp honey
- 1 tbsp olive oil
- 1/2 tsp dried thyme
- Salt and pepper to taste
- Lemon wedges, for serving

Prep Time: 10 min

Cook Time: 15 min

Serves: 4

Directions

1. Preheat the oven to 400°F (200°C). Line a baking sheet with parchment paper or lightly grease it.

2. In a small bowl, mix together the chopped walnuts, dried thyme, salt, and pepper.

3. In another small bowl, whisk together the Dijon mustard, honey, and olive oil.

4. Place the salmon fillets on the prepared baking sheet. Brush the mustard-honey mixture evenly over the top of each fillet.

5. Press the walnut mixture onto the mustard-coated side of each salmon fillet, forming a crust.

6. Bake in the preheated oven for 12-15 minutes, or until the salmon is cooked through and the walnut crust is golden brown and crispy.

7. Serve the salmon fillets hot, garnished with lemon wedges.

Nutritional Information: Calories: 330, Protein: 30g, Carbohydrates: 8g, Fat: 20g, Fiber: 2g, Cholesterol: 70mg, Sodium: 250mg

Scallops Seared with Garlic and Basil

Ingredients

- 1 pound fresh scallops
- 2 tbsp olive oil
- 4 cloves garlic, minced
- 1/4 cup fresh basil leaves, chopped
- Salt and pepper to taste

Prep Time: 10 min

Cook Time: 5 min

Serves: 4

Directions

1. Pat the scallops dry with paper towels and season them with salt and pepper.

2. Heat the olive oil in a large skillet over medium-high heat.

3. Add the minced garlic to the skillet and sauté for 1-2 minutes until fragrant.

4. Carefully add the scallops to the skillet in a single layer, making sure not to overcrowd them. Cook for 2-3 minutes on each side until golden brown and cooked through.

5. Sprinkle the chopped basil over the scallops and cook for an additional 30 seconds to 1 minute.

6. Remove the skillet from the heat and serve the scallops immediately over preferred side, garnished with additional fresh basil if desired.

Nutritional Information: Calories: 180, Protein: 25g, Carbohydrates: 2g, Fat: 8g, Fiber: 0g, Cholesterol: 40mg, Sodium: 350mg

Pesto Rubbed Halibut with Roasted Tomatoes

 Prep Time: 15 min   Cook Time: 20 min   Serves: 4

Ingredients

- 4 halibut fillets (about 6 oz each)
- Salt and pepper to taste
- 2 cups cherry tomatoes
- 2 tbsp olive oil

For Pesto:
- 2 cups fresh basil leaves
- 1/4 cup pine nuts
- 2 cloves garlic
- 1/2 cup grated Parmesan cheese
- 1/2 cup extra virgin olive oil
- Salt and pepper to taste

Directions

1. Make the Pesto (or use store-bought): In a food processor, combine the basil leaves, pine nuts, and garlic. Pulse until finely chopped.

2. Add the Parmesan cheese and pulse again until combined.

3. With the food processor running, slowly drizzle in the olive oil until the pesto reaches your desired consistency. Season with salt and pepper to taste.

4. Prepare the Halibut: Preheat the oven to 400°F (200°C). Season the halibut fillets with salt and pepper, then rub each fillet with a generous amount of pesto.

5. Place the halibut fillets on a baking sheet lined with parchment paper. Arrange the cherry tomatoes around the fillets and drizzle them with olive oil.

6. Roast in the preheated oven for 15-20 minutes, or until the halibut is cooked through and flakes easily with a fork, and the tomatoes are blistered and juicy.

7. Serve the pesto-rubbed halibut alongside the roasted tomatoes, and garnish with additional fresh basil leaves if desired.

Nutritional Information: Calories: 380, Protein: 32g, Carbohydrates: 5g, Fat: 27g, Fiber: 2g, Cholesterol: 70mg, Sodium: 270mg

Macadamia Cod with Mango-Mint Salsa

 Prep Time: 15 min   Cook Time: 15 min   Serves: 4

Ingredients

- 4 cod fillets (about 6 oz each)
- 1 cup macadamia nuts, finely chopped
- 1/4 cup fresh parsley, chopped
- 1 tsp garlic powder
- 1/2 tsp paprika
- Salt and pepper, to taste
- 2 eggs, beaten
- 2 tbsp olive oil

For Mango-Mint Salsa:
- 2 ripe mangoes, diced
- 1/4 cup red onion, finely chopped
- 1/4 cup fresh mint leaves, chopped
- 1 jalapeño, seeded and minced
- Juice of 1 lime
- Salt and pepper, to taste

Directions

1. Preheat the oven to 400°F (200°C). Line a baking sheet with parchment paper.

2. In a shallow dish, combine the chopped macadamia nuts, chopped parsley, garlic powder, paprika, salt, and pepper.

3. Dip each cod fillet into the beaten eggs, then coat it with the macadamia mixture, pressing gently to adhere. Place the coated fillets on the prepared baking sheet.

4. Drizzle the cod fillets with olive oil and bake in the preheated oven for 12-15 minutes, or until the fish flakes easily with a fork and the crust is golden brown.

5. While the cod is baking, prepare the mango-mint salsa. In a bowl, combine the diced mangoes, red onion, chopped mint leaves, minced jalapeño, lime juice, salt, and pepper. Stir well to combine.

6. Serve the baked cod fillets hot, topped with the mango-mint salsa.

Nutritional Information: Calories: 420, Protein: 30g, Carbohydrates: 20g, Fat: 25g, Fiber: 5g, Cholesterol: 85mg, Sodium: 350mg

Peppercorn Mackerel with Horseradish Sauce

 Prep Time: 10 min   Cook Time: 15 min   Serves: 4

Ingredients

- 4 mackerel fillets
- 2 tbsp whole peppercorns
- 1 tbsp olive oil
- Salt, to taste
- 1/4 cup Greek yogurt
- 2 tbsp prepared horseradish
- 1 tbsp lemon juice
- 1 tbsp chopped fresh dill
- Lemon wedges, for serving

Directions

1. Preheat the oven to 400°F (200°C). Line a baking sheet with parchment paper.

2. Place the peppercorns in a mortar and pestle or spice grinder and crush them until coarsely ground.

3. Rub the crushed peppercorns onto both sides of the mackerel fillets. Season with salt.

4. Heat the olive oil in a skillet over medium-high heat. Add the mackerel fillets and cook for 2-3 minutes on each side, or until golden brown and cooked through.

5. While the mackerel is cooking, prepare the horseradish sauce. In a small bowl, combine the Greek yogurt, horseradish, lemon juice, and chopped dill. Mix well.

6. Once the mackerel is cooked, transfer it to the prepared baking sheet and place it in the oven for 5 minutes to finish cooking.

7. Serve the peppercorn-crusted mackerel hot with a dollop of horseradish sauce and lemon wedges on the side.

Nutritional Information: Calories: 280, Protein: 25g, Carbohydrates: 2g, Fat: 18g, Fiber: 1g, Cholesterol: 90mg, Sodium: 300mg

Grilled Trout with Almond Parsley Pesto

 Prep Time: 15 min   Cook Time: 15 min   Serves: 4

Ingredients

- 4 trout fillets
- 2 tbsp olive oil
- Salt and pepper to taste
- 1 cup fresh parsley leaves
- 1/2 cup almonds
- 2 cloves garlic
- 1/4 cup grated Parmesan cheese
- 1/4 cup olive oil (for pesto)
- 1 tbsp lemon juice

Directions

1. Preheat grill to medium-high heat. Brush trout fillets with 2 tbsp olive oil and season with salt and pepper.

2. Place trout fillets on the grill, skin side down. Grill for 5-7 minutes per side or until fish flakes easily with a fork.

3. In a food processor, combine parsley, almonds, garlic, Parmesan cheese, and lemon juice. Pulse until finely chopped.

4. With the processor running, slowly add 1/4 cup olive oil until the mixture becomes smooth. Serve the grilled trout topped with the almond parsley pesto.

Nutritional Information: Calories: 420, Protein: 32g, Carbohydrates: 5g, Fat: 30g, Fiber: 3g, Cholesterol: 80mg, Sodium: 220mg

Chapter 7: Poultry

Grilled Chicken with Avocado Salsa

 Prep Time: 10 min   Cook Time: 25 min   Serves: 4

Ingredients

- 4 boneless, skinless chicken breasts
- 1 tbsp olive oil
- 1 tsp paprika
- 1 tsp garlic powder
- Salt and pepper to taste

For Avocado Salsa:
- 2 ripe avocados, diced
- 1 tomato, diced
- 1/4 cup red onion, finely chopped
- 1/4 cup fresh cilantro, chopped
- Juice of 1 lime

Directions

1. Preheat the grill to medium-high heat.
2. In a small bowl, mix together the olive oil, paprika, garlic powder, salt, and pepper. Brush the chicken breasts with the olive oil mixture.
3. Grill the chicken breasts for 6-7 minutes on each side, or until cooked through and no longer pink in the center.
4. While the chicken is grilling, prepare the avocado salsa. In a medium bowl, combine the diced avocados, tomato, red onion, cilantro, lime juice, salt, and pepper. Mix well to combine.
5. Once the chicken is cooked, remove it from the grill and let it rest for a few minutes. Serve the grilled chicken topped with the avocado salsa.

Nutritional Information: Calories: 320, Protein: 25g, Carbohydrates: 10g, Fat: 20g, Fiber: 6g, Cholesterol: 80mg, Sodium: 350mg

Turmeric Chicken Skewers

 Prep Time: 15 min   Cook Time: 12 min   Serves: 4

Ingredients

- 1 lb chicken breast, cut into cubes
- 1/4 cup plain yogurt
- 2 tbsp olive oil
- 1 tbsp lemon juice
- 2 tsp turmeric powder
- 1 tsp cumin powder
- 1 tsp paprika
- 1/2 tsp garlic powder
- 1/2 tsp ground ginger
- Salt and pepper to taste
- Wooden or metal skewers, soaked if wooden

Directions

1. In a bowl, mix together the yogurt, olive oil, lemon juice, turmeric, cumin, paprika, garlic powder, ginger, salt, and pepper to create the marinade.
2. Add the cubed chicken to the marinade, making sure each piece is well coated. Cover and refrigerate for at least 1 hour, or overnight for best flavor.
3. Preheat the grill or grill pan over medium-high heat. If using wooden skewers, make sure to soak them in water for at least 30 minutes to prevent burning.
4. Thread the marinated chicken onto the skewers, dividing evenly.
5. Grill the skewers for about 5-6 minutes on each side, or until the chicken is cooked through and slightly charred.
6. Serve the turmeric chicken skewers hot, optionally garnished with fresh herbs or a squeeze of lemon.

Nutritional Information: Calories: 230, Protein: 28g, Carbohydrates: 2g, Fat: 12g, Fiber: 1g, Cholesterol: 80mg, Sodium: 330mg

Chicken and Spinach Curry

 Prep Time: 10 min   Cook Time: 25 min   Serves: 4

Ingredients

- 1 tbsp olive oil
- 1 onion, diced
- 2 cloves garlic, minced
- 1 tbsp ginger, minced
- 1 pound chicken breast, cut into bite-sized pieces
- 2 tbsp curry powder
- 1 tsp turmeric powder
- 1 tsp cumin powder
- 1 tsp coriander powder
- 1/2 tsp cayenne pepper
- 1 can (14 oz) diced tomatoes
- 1 can (14 oz) coconut milk (or 1 cup plain Greek yogurt)
- 4 cups fresh spinach leaves
- Salt and pepper to taste
- Fresh cilantro for garnish (optional)

Directions

1. Heat the olive oil in a large skillet over medium heat. Add the diced onion and cook until translucent, about 3-4 minutes.

2. Add the minced garlic and ginger to the skillet, and cook for another 1-2 minutes until fragrant.

3. Add the chicken pieces to the skillet and cook until browned on all sides, about 5-6 minutes.

4. Stir in the curry powder, turmeric, cumin, coriander, and cayenne pepper until the chicken is evenly coated with the spices.

5. Pour in the diced tomatoes and coconut milk (or yogurt). Bring the mixture to a simmer, then reduce the heat to low and let it cook for 10-15 minutes, stirring occasionally, until the chicken is cooked through and the sauce has thickened slightly.

6. Stir in the fresh spinach leaves and let them wilt into the curry. Season with salt and pepper to taste.

7. Serve the chicken and spinach curry hot over cooked rice or quinoa. Garnish with fresh cilantro if desired.

Nutritional Information: Calories: 350, Protein: 30g, Carbohydrates: 15g, Fat: 20g, Fiber: 5g, Cholesterol: 80mg, Sodium: 600mg

Spiced Chicken Shawarma Wraps

 Prep Time: 15 min   Cook Time: 15 min   Serves: 4

Ingredients

- 1 lb boneless, skinless chicken breasts, thinly sliced
- 2 tbsp olive oil
- 2 cloves garlic, minced
- 1 tsp cumin powder
- 1 tsp paprika powder
- 1/2 tsp turmeric powder
- 1/2 tsp coriander powder
- 1/4 tsp cinnamon powder
- Salt and black pepper to taste
- 4 gluten-free tortillas
- 1 cup shredded lettuce or arugula
- 1 cup diced tomatoes
- 1/2 cup diced cucumbers
- 1/4 cup chopped fresh parsley
- Tahini sauce for serving

Directions

1. In a bowl, combine the olive oil, minced garlic, cumin, paprika, turmeric, coriander, cinnamon, salt, and black pepper. Add the sliced chicken breasts and toss until well coated. Let marinate for at least 10 minutes.

2. Heat a skillet over medium-high heat. Add the marinated chicken and cook for 5-7 minutes, or until cooked through and slightly charred.

3. Warm the gluten-free tortillas according to package instructions.

4. Assemble the wraps: Place a spoonful of cooked chicken on each tortilla. Top with shredded lettuce or arugula, diced tomatoes, diced cucumbers, and chopped fresh parsley. Drizzle with tahini sauce.

5. Roll up the wraps, tucking in the sides as you go, and secure with toothpicks if necessary.

Nutritional Information: Calories: 320, Protein: 25g, Carbohydrates: 20g, Fat: 15g, Fiber: 3g, Cholesterol: 70mg, Sodium: 480mg

Spinach and Feta Stuffed Chicken Breasts

Prep Time: 15 min   Cook Time: 25 min   Serves: 4

Ingredients

- 4 boneless, skinless chicken breasts
- 2 cups fresh spinach, chopped
- 1/2 cup crumbled feta cheese
- 1 tsp garlic powder
- Salt and pepper to taste
- 1 tbsp olive oil
- 1 cup plain Greek yogurt
- 1/2 tsp turmeric powder
- 1/2 tsp cumin powder
- 1/2 tsp paprika
- Fresh parsley for garnish (optional)

Directions

1. Preheat the oven to 375°F (190°C).
2. In a mixing bowl, combine the chopped spinach, crumbled feta cheese, garlic powder, salt, and pepper.
3. Using a sharp knife, cut a pocket into each chicken breast, being careful not to cut all the way through. Stuff each chicken breast with the spinach and feta mixture, then secure with toothpicks if needed to keep the filling in place.
4. Heat olive oil in a large oven-safe skillet over medium-high heat. Add the stuffed chicken breasts and cook for 3-4 minutes on each side, or until golden brown.
5. In a small bowl, mix together the Greek yogurt, cumin, turmeric, and paprika until well combined. Pour the yogurt sauce over the chicken breasts in the skillet.
6. Transfer the skillet to the preheated oven and bake for 15-20 minutes, or until the chicken is cooked through and reaches an internal temperature of 165°F (75°C).
7. Remove the toothpicks from the chicken breasts before serving. Garnish with fresh parsley if desired.

Nutritional Information: Calories: 280, Protein: 35g, Carbohydrates: 5g, Fat: 12g, Fiber: 1g, Cholesterol: 90mg, Sodium: 320mg

Healing Spice Chicken with Apricots

Prep Time: 15 min   Cook Time: 45 min   Serves: 4

Ingredients

- 4 bone-in, skinless chicken thighs
- 1 tbsp olive oil
- 1 onion, chopped
- 3 cloves garlic, minced
- 1 tsp cumin powder
- 1 tsp coriander powder
- 1/2 tsp cinnamon powder
- 1/2 tsp ground ginger
- 1/4 tsp turmeric powder
- 1/4 tsp ground paprika
- 1/4 tsp ground cayenne pepper
- 1 cup low-sodium chicken broth
- 1/2 cup dried apricots, chopped
- 1/4 cup green olives, pitted
- Salt and pepper,
- Fresh cilantro or parsley, for garnish

Directions

1. Season the chicken thighs with salt and pepper. In a large skillet or tagine, heat the olive oil over medium heat. Add the chicken thighs and brown on both sides, about 5 minutes per side. Remove the chicken from the skillet and set aside.
2. In the same skillet, cook chopped onion until softened, about 5 minutes. Add the minced garlic and cook for an additional 1-2 minutes.
3. Stir in the cumin, coriander, cinnamon, ginger, turmeric, paprika, and cayenne pepper (if using). Cook for 1 minute, stirring constantly, until fragrant.
4. Return the chicken thighs to the skillet. Add the chicken broth and dried apricots. Bring to a simmer, then reduce the heat to low. Cover and cook for 30 minutes, or until the chicken is cooked through and tender.
5. Stir in the green olives and cook for an additional 5 minutes. Taste and adjust seasoning with salt and pepper if needed. Serve over quinoa or rice. Garnish with fresh cilantro or parsley.

Nutritional Information: Calories: 330, Protein: 24g, Carbohydrates: 18g, Fat: 16g, Fiber: 3g, Cholesterol: 70mg, Sodium: 430mg

Barbecue Chicken Tenders

Prep Time: 15 min Cook Time: 20 min Serves: 4

Ingredients

- 1 lb boneless, skinless chicken breasts, cut into strips
- 1 cup almond flour
- 1/2 cup unsweetened shredded coconut
- 1 tsp garlic powder
- 1 tsp paprika
- 1/2 tsp salt
- 1/4 tsp black pepper
- 2 eggs, beaten
- Cooking spray or olive oil

For Barbecue Sauce:

- 1 cup tomato sauce
- 2 tbsp apple cider vinegar
- 1 tbsp coconut aminos
- 1 tbsp Dijon mustard
- 1 tbsp smoked paprika
- 1 tsp garlic powder
- 1 tsp onion powder
- 1/2 tsp ground black pepper
- Pinch of cayenne pepper

Directions

1. Preheat the oven to 400°F (200°C). Line a baking sheet with parchment paper and lightly coat it with olive oil.

2. In a shallow dish, combine the almond flour, shredded coconut, garlic powder, paprika, salt and black pepper.

3. Dip each chicken strip into the beaten eggs, then coat it evenly with the almond flour mixture. Place the coated chicken strips on the prepared baking sheet.

4. Bake for 18-20 minutes, or until the chicken is cooked through and the coating is golden brown and crispy.

5. In a small saucepan, combine all the ingredients for the barbecue sauce.

6. Bring the mixture to a simmer over medium heat, then reduce the heat to low.

7. Cook the sauce, stirring occasionally, for 10-15 minutes, or until it thickens slightly. Remove the sauce from the heat and let it cool before serving.

Nutritional Information: Calories: 280, Protein: 25g, Carbohydrates: 2g, Fat: 18g, Fiber: 1g, Cholesterol: 90mg, Sodium: 300mg

Ground Turkey Stuffed Bell Peppers

Prep Time: 15 min Cook Time: 30 min Serves: 4

Ingredients

- 4 large bell peppers, tops cut off and seeds removed
- 1 tbsp olive oil
- 1 pound ground turkey
- 1 onion, chopped
- 2 cloves garlic, minced
- 1 cup spinach, chopped
- 1 tsp dried oregano
- 1/2 tsp salt
- 1/4 tsp black pepper
- 1/2 cup cooked quinoa or brown rice
- 1/2 cup low-sodium tomato sauce
- 1/4 cup grated Parmesan cheese (optional or omit for dairy-free option)

Directions

1. Preheat oven to 375°F (190°C). Place the bell peppers upright in a baking dish; set aside.

2. Heat olive oil in a skillet over medium heat. Add ground turkey, onion, and garlic, and cook until the turkey is browned and onions are soft.

3. Stir in spinach, oregano, salt, pepper, and cook until the spinach is wilted.

4. Remove from heat and mix in the cooked quinoa or brown rice and half of the tomato sauce.

5. Spoon the turkey mixture into each bell pepper. Top with the remaining tomato sauce and optional Parmesan cheese.

6. Cover with parchment paper and bake for 25-30 minutes, or until the peppers are tender.

Nutritional Information: Calories: 290, Protein: 27g, Carbohydrates: 21g, Fat: 11g, Fiber: 4g, Cholesterol: 80mg, Sodium: 320mg

Cauliflower Chicken Fajita Bowls

Prep Time: 15 min   Cook Time: 30 min   Serves: 4

Ingredients

- 1 lb chicken breast, thinly sliced
- 2 bell peppers, sliced
- 1 onion, sliced
- 2 tbsp olive oil
- 1 tsp chili powder
- 1 tsp cumin
- Salt and pepper, to taste

- 1/2 tsp paprika
- 2 avocados, sliced
- 4 cups cauliflower rice (fresh or frozen)
- Lime wedges, for serving
- Fresh cilantro, for garnish

Directions

1. In a large skillet, heat 1 tablespoon of olive oil over medium-high heat. Add the sliced chicken breast and season with chili powder, cumin, paprika, salt, and pepper. Cook for 5-7 minutes, or until the chicken is cooked through. Remove from the skillet and set aside.

2. In the same skillet, add the remaining tablespoon of olive oil. Add the sliced bell peppers and onion. Cook for 5-6 minutes, or until the vegetables are tender and slightly caramelized.

3. While the vegetables are cooking, prepare the cauliflower rice according to package instructions. If using fresh cauliflower rice, you can sauté it in a separate skillet with a little olive oil until tender.

4. To assemble the bowls, divide the cauliflower rice among serving bowls. Top with the cooked chicken, bell peppers, and onions. Add sliced avocado on top.

5. Garnish with fresh cilantro and serve with lime wedges for squeezing over the bowls.

Nutritional Information: Calories: 320, Protein: 25g, Carbohydrates: 15g, Fat: 18g, Fiber: 7g, Cholesterol: 80mg, Sodium: 480mg

Rustic Chicken with Peppers

Prep Time: 15 min   Cook Time: 45 min   Serves: 4

Ingredients

- 4 bone-in, skinless chicken thighs
- Salt and pepper, to taste
- 2 tbsp olive oil
- 1 onion, chopped
- 2 cloves garlic, minced
- 1 red bell pepper, sliced
- 1 yellow bell pepper, sliced

- 1 can (14 oz) diced tomatoes
- 1/2 cup chicken broth
- 1 tsp dried oregano
- 1 tsp dried basil
- 1/2 cup pitted olives (green or black), sliced
- Fresh parsley, chopped, for garnish

Directions

1. Season the chicken thighs with salt and pepper.

2. In a large skillet, heat the olive oil over medium-high heat. Add the chicken thighs and cook until browned on both sides, about 5 minutes per side. Remove the chicken from the skillet and set aside.

3. In the same skillet, add the chopped onion and cook until softened, about 3 minutes. Add the minced garlic and cook for another minute.

4. Add the sliced bell peppers to the skillet and cook for 5 minutes, or until they start to soften.

5. Stir in the diced tomatoes, chicken broth, dried oregano, and dried basil. Return the chicken thighs to the skillet, nestling them into the sauce. Cover and simmer for 25-30 minutes, or until the chicken is cooked through.

6. Stir in the sliced olives and cook for another 5 minutes. Adjust seasoning with salt and pepper if needed.

7. Garnish with fresh parsley before serving.

Nutritional Information: Calories: 320, Protein: 25g, Carbohydrates: 10g, Fat: 20g, Fiber: 3g, Cholesterol: 80mg, Sodium: 600mg

Duck Breast in Tart Cherry Sauce

Prep Time: 10 min   Cook Time: 20 min   Serves: 4

Ingredients

- 4 duck breast fillets
- Salt and pepper to taste
- 1 tbsp olive oil
- 1 cup tart cherry juice concentrate
- 2 tbsp balsamic vinegar
- 1 tbsp honey
- 1 tsp ground flaxseeds or rice flour (optional, for thickening)
- Fresh parsley for garnish (optional)

Directions

1. Score the skin of the duck breast fillets with a sharp knife, being careful not to cut into the meat. Season both sides of the duck breasts generously with salt and pepper.

2. Heat a large skillet over medium-high heat. Add the olive oil to the skillet.

3. Place the duck breasts skin side down in the skillet. Cook for 6-8 minutes, or until the skin is crispy and golden brown. Flip the duck breasts and continue cooking for another 4-6 minutes, or until cooked to your desired level of doneness. Remove the duck breasts from the skillet and set aside to rest.

4. In the same skillet, reduce the heat to medium. Add the tart cherry juice concentrate, balsamic vinegar, and honey. Stir to combine, scraping up any browned bits from the bottom of the skillet. Simmer for 5-7 minutes, or until the sauce has thickened slightly.

5. If desired, you can thicken the sauce further by whisking in ground flaxseeds or rice flour. Continue simmering for another 2-3 minutes.

6. Slice the rested duck breasts and serve drizzled with the cherry sauce. Serve over your preferred side. Garnish with fresh parsley if desired.

Nutritional Information: Calories: 350, Protein: 25g, Carbohydrates: 15g, Fat: 20g, Fiber: 1g, Cholesterol: 85mg, Sodium: 100mg

BBQ Grilled Chicken with Peach Salsa

Prep Time: 15 min   Cook Time: 20 min   Serves: 4

Ingredients

- 4 boneless, skinless chicken breasts
- 2 medium zucchinis, sliced lengthwise
- 2 peaches, diced
- 1/4 cup red onion, finely chopped
- 2 tbsp fresh cilantro, chopped
- 1/4 cup olive oil
- 1/2 tbsp BBQ spice blend
- 2 limes
- 1 tbsp of honey
- Salt and pepper to taste

Directions

1. Preheat your grill to medium-high heat.

2. Pat chicken dry and season all over with BBQ spice blend and a pinch each of salt and pepper, then brush them with olive oil.

3. Place the chicken breasts on the grill and cook for 6-8 minutes per side, or until they are cooked through and have grill marks.

4. While the chicken is cooking, place the sliced zucchinis on the grill and cook for 3-4 minutes per side, until they are tender and have grill marks.

5. In a bowl, combine chopped cilantro, zest and juice of 1 lime, cut remaining lime into wedges. Whisk in all of the honey and olive oil; season to taste with salt and pepper. Stir in chopped cilantro, diced peaches, and red onion.

6. Once the chicken and zucchini are cooked, remove them from the grill and serve with lime wedges and peach salsa on top.

Nutritional Information: Calories: 320, Protein: 30g, Carbohydrates: 15g, Fat: 12g, Fiber: 4g, Cholesterol: 75mg, Sodium: 400mg

Roasted Chicken with Root Vegetables

 Prep Time: 15 min   Cook Time: 45 min   Serves: 4

Ingredients

- 4 bone-in, skin-on chicken thighs
- 3 medium carrots, peeled and chopped
- 2 parsnips, peeled and chopped
- 1 large sweet potato, peeled and chopped
- 2 tbsp olive oil
- 2 cloves garlic, minced
- 1 tsp dried thyme
- Salt and pepper to taste
- Fresh parsley for garnish (optional)

Directions

1. Preheat your oven to 400°F (200°C). Line a baking sheet with parchment paper for easy cleanup.

2. In a large bowl, toss the chopped carrots, parsnips, and sweet potatoes with olive oil, minced garlic, dried thyme, salt, and pepper until evenly coated.

3. Place the chicken thighs on the prepared baking sheet and arrange the seasoned root vegetables around them.

4. Roast in the preheated oven for 35-45 minutes, or until the chicken is cooked through (internal temperature of 165°F/75°C) and the vegetables are tender, stirring the vegetables halfway through cooking.

5. Once done, remove from the oven and let the chicken rest for a few minutes before serving. Garnish with fresh parsley if desired.

Nutritional Information: Calories: 380, Protein: 25g, Carbohydrates: 20g, Fat: 22g, Fiber: 5g, Cholesterol: 120mg, Sodium: 380mg

Coconut Lime Chicken with Cauliflower Rice

 Prep Time: 15 min   Cook Time: 30 min   Serves: 4

Ingredients

For Coconut Lime Chicken:
- 4 boneless, skinless chicken breasts
- 1 can (13.5 oz) coconut milk
- 2 limes, zested and juiced
- 2 cloves garlic, minced
- 1 tsp cumin powder
- 1 tsp coriander powder
- 1/2 tsp turmeric powder
- 1 tsp salt
- 1/2 tsp black pepper

For Cauliflower Rice:
- 1 large head of cauliflower, cut into florets
- 2 tbsp coconut oil
- 1 small onion, finely chopped
- 2 cloves garlic, minced
- 1/4 tsp salt
- 1/4 tsp black pepper
- 1/4 cup fresh cilantro, chopped
- Juice of 1 lime

Directions

1. Combine coconut milk, lime zest, lime juice, garlic, cumin, coriander, turmeric, salt, and pepper. Add and marinate chicken for at least 30 minutes.

2. Heat 1 tablespoon coconut oil in a skillet over medium-high heat. Cook chicken for 6-7 minutes on each side, until internal temperature reaches 165°F (74°C). Remove chicken and set aside.

3. Pulse cauliflower florets in a food processor until rice-sized.

4. Heat 1 tablespoon coconut oil in a skillet over medium heat. Sauté onion for 3-4 minutes, add garlic for 1 minute, then add cauliflower rice, salt, and pepper. Cook for 5-7 minutes, stirring occasionally, until tender.

5. Stir lime juice and cilantro into the cauliflower rice. Serve chicken over cauliflower rice, garnished with more cilantro if desired.

Nutritional Information: Calories: 450, Protein: 38g, Carbohydrates: 16g, Fat: 29g, Fiber: 6g, Cholesterol: 80mg, Sodium: 620mg

Turkey Meatballs with Zucchini Noodles

Ingredients

- 1 pound ground turkey
- 1/4 cup almond flour
- 1/4 cup grated Parmesan cheese
- 1 egg
- 2 cloves garlic, minced
- 1 tsp dried oregano
- 1/2 tsp dried basil
- Salt and pepper to taste
- 4 medium zucchinis, spiralized into noodles
- Fresh basil leaves, for garnish

For the Marinara Sauce (if store-bought use 2 cups):

- 1 tbsp olive oil
- 1 onion, diced
- 2 cloves garlic, minced
- 1 can (14 oz) crushed tomatoes
- 1 tsp dried oregano
- 1 tsp dried basil
- Salt and pepper to taste

Prep Time: 15 min   Cook Time: 25-35 min   Serves: 4

Directions

1. Preheat the oven to 400°F (200°C). Line a baking sheet with parchment paper or lightly grease it.

2. In a large bowl, combine the ground turkey, almond flour, Parmesan cheese, egg, minced garlic, dried oregano, dried basil, salt, and pepper. Mix until well combined.

3. Roll the turkey mixture into meatballs, about 1 inch in diameter, and place them on the prepared baking sheet.

4. Bake the meatballs in the preheated oven for 15-20 minutes, or until cooked through and golden brown.

5. While the meatballs are baking, spiralize the zucchinis into noodles using a spiralizer.

6. In a large skillet, heat olive oil in a large skillet over medium heat. Add diced onion and cook until softened, about 5 minutes. Add minced garlic and cook for an additional minute. Stir in crushed tomatoes, dried oregano, dried basil, salt, and pepper. Bring the sauce to a simmer and let it cook for 10-15 minutes, stirring occasionally.

7. If store-bought, in a large skillet heat the marinara sauce over medium heat.

8. Once heated, add the zucchini noodles and cook for 3-4 minutes, or until the noodles are tender.

9. Serve the turkey meatballs over the zucchini noodles, garnished with fresh basil leaves.

Nutritional Information: Calories: 350, Protein: 30g, Carbohydrates: 12g, Fat: 20g, Fiber: 4g, Cholesterol: 120mg, Sodium: 680mg

 PRO TIP:

For extra dose of veggies and to keep turkey meatballs moist and tender add 1 cup of grated zucchini, juices squeezed, to the meatball mix. Grated carrots or finely chopped spinach would also work well, or mix all three for even more benefits.

Zesty Ginger Detox Chicken

 Prep Time: 15 min Cook Time: 25 min Serves: 4

Ingredients

- 4 boneless, skinless chicken breasts
- 1 cup plain Greek yogurt
- 2 tbsp lemon juice
- 2 tbsp olive oil
- 2 cloves garlic, minced
- 1 tbsp fresh ginger, grated
- 1 tsp turmeric powder
- 1 tsp cumin powder
- 1 tsp coriander powder
- 1 tsp paprika
- 1 tsp cinnamon powder
- 1 tsp ground black pepper
- 1 tsp sea salt
- 1/2 tsp cayenne pepper
- Fresh cilantro, chopped

Directions

1. In a large bowl, mix together the Greek yogurt, lemon juice, olive oil, garlic, ginger, turmeric, cumin, coriander, paprika, cinnamon, black pepper, sea salt, and cayenne pepper (if using).

2. Add the chicken breasts to the bowl, coating them thoroughly with the marinade. Cover and refrigerate for at least 1 hour, preferably overnight for best results.

3. Preheat the oven to 400°F (200°C). Place the marinated chicken breasts on a baking sheet lined with parchment paper.

4. Bake the chicken for 20-25 minutes, or until fully cooked and the internal temperature reaches 165°F (74°C). Garnish with fresh cilantro before serving.

Nutritional Information: Calories: 300, Protein: 35g, Carbohydrates: 5g, Fat: 15g, Fiber: 2g, Cholesterol: 90mg, Sodium: 450mg

Golden Curry Chicken Skewers

 Prep Time: 20 min Cook Time: 15 min Serves: 4

Ingredients

- 1 lb boneless, skinless chicken breasts, cut into 1-inch cubes
- 1 cup coconut milk
- 1 tsp turmeric powder
- 1 tsp curry powder
- 1 tbsp honey
- 2 cloves garlic, minced
- 1 tbsp fresh ginger, grated
- 1 tbsp olive oil
- Salt and pepper to taste
- Wooden skewers, soaked in water for 30 minutes

Directions

1. In a large bowl, mix coconut milk, turmeric powder, curry powder, honey, minced garlic, grated ginger, olive oil, salt, and pepper. Add chicken cubes and toss to coat. Marinate for at least 1 hour in the refrigerator.

2. Preheat grill to medium-high heat. Thread marinated chicken onto soaked skewers.

3. Grill chicken skewers for about 12-15 minutes, turning occasionally, until chicken is cooked through and has nice grill marks.

4. Serve hot with a side of your favorite anti-inflammatory vegetables or a fresh salad.

Nutritional Information: Calories: 320, Protein: 25g, Carbohydrates: 10g, Fat: 22g, Fiber: 2g, Cholesterol: 70mg, Sodium: 250mg

Supercharged Chicken and Veggie Stir-Fry

Ingredients

- 1 lb boneless, skinless chicken breast, thinly sliced
- 2 cups broccoli florets
- 2 cups cauliflower florets
- 1 cup sliced carrots
- 1 cup sweet peas
- 2 tbsp olive oil
- 4 cloves garlic, minced
- 1 tbsp grated fresh ginger
- 1/4 cup low-sodium soy sauce or tamari
- 2 tbsp rice vinegar
- 1 tbsp honey or maple syrup (optional)
- 1 tbsp ground flax seeds or rice flour (optional)
- Sesame seeds and chopped green onions for garnish
- Salt and pepper to taste

Prep Time: 15 min   Cook Time: 15 min   Serves: 4

Directions

1. In a small bowl, whisk together the soy sauce, rice vinegar, and honey or maple syrup if using. Set aside.

2. Heat 1 tablespoon of olive oil in a large skillet or wok over medium-high heat. Add the chicken slices and stir-fry until cooked through, about 5-6 minutes. Remove the chicken from the skillet and set aside.

3. In the same skillet, add the remaining tablespoon of olive oil. Add the minced garlic and grated ginger, and stir-fry for 1-2 minutes until fragrant.

4. Add the broccoli, cauliflower, carrots, and sweet peas to the skillet. Stir-fry for 5-6 minutes until the vegetables are tender-crisp.

5. Return the cooked chicken to the skillet. Pour the soy sauce mixture over the chicken and vegetables, and toss everything together until well coated. If desired, add ground flax seeds or rice flour dissolved in 2 tablespoons of water to the skillet to thicken the sauce.

6. Cook for an additional 2-3 minutes, stirring constantly, until the sauce has thickened and everything is heated through.

7. Season with salt and pepper to taste. Garnish with sesame seeds and chopped green onions if desired.

Nutritional Information: Calories: 350, Protein: 30g, Carbohydrates: 12g, Fat: 20g, Fiber: 4g, Cholesterol: 120mg, Sodium: 680mg

Baked Lemon Pepper Chicken

Ingredients

- 4 boneless, skinless chicken breasts
- 2 tbsp olive oil
- 1 lemon (zested and juiced)
- 2 tsp freshly ground black pepper
- 1 tsp sea salt
- 2 cloves garlic (minced)
- 1 tsp dried thyme
- 1 tsp dried rosemary

Prep Time: 10 min   Cook Time: 30 min   Serves: 4

Directions

1. Preheat your oven to 400°F (200°C) and line a baking dish with parchment paper.

2. In a small bowl, combine olive oil, lemon zest, lemon juice, black pepper, sea salt, minced garlic, dried thyme, and dried rosemary.

3. Place the chicken breasts in the baking dish and coat them evenly with the lemon pepper mixture.

4. Bake in the preheated oven for 25-30 minutes, or until the chicken reaches an internal temperature of 165°F (75°C) and the juices run clear.

Nutritional Information: Calories: 250, Protein: 30g, Carbohydrates: 2g, Fat: 12g, Fiber: 1g, Cholesterol: 75mg, Sodium: 400mg

Chicken Casserole with Artichokes

Prep Time: 15 min   **Cook Time: 25 min**   **Serves: 4**

Ingredients

- 1 cup quinoa, rinsed
- 2 1/2 cups chicken broth
- 4 boneless, skinless chicken breasts
- Salt and pepper to taste
- 2 tbsp olive oil
- 3 cloves garlic, minced
- 1/4 cup lemon juice
- Zest of 1 lemon
- 1/4 cup capers, drained
- 1 can (14 oz) artichoke hearts, drained and chopped
- 2 tbsp chopped fresh parsley
- 1/4 cup grated Parmesan cheese (optional)

Directions

1. Preheat your oven to 375°F (190°C). Lightly grease a 9x13-inch baking dish.

2. In a medium saucepan, combine the quinoa and 2 cups of chicken broth. Bring to a boil, then reduce heat to low, cover, and simmer for about 15 minutes, or until the quinoa is cooked and the liquid is absorbed.

3. While the quinoa is cooking, season the chicken breasts with salt and pepper. In a large skillet, heat the olive oil over medium-high heat. Add the chicken breasts and cook for 4-5 minutes on each side, or until golden brown and cooked through. Remove the chicken from the skillet and set aside.

4. In the same skillet, add the minced garlic and cook for 1 minute, until fragrant. Add the lemon juice and ½ cup of chicken broth, scraping up any browned bits from the bottom of the skillet.

5. Stir in the capers and chopped artichoke hearts. Cook for 2-3 minutes, allowing the flavors to meld together.

6. Place the cooked quinoa in the prepared baking dish. Arrange the cooked chicken breasts on top of the quinoa. Pour the caper and artichoke mixture over the chicken.

7. Sprinkle the lemon zest, chopped parsley and grated Parmesan cheese, if using over the top of the casserole.

8. Bake in the preheated oven for 15-20 minutes, or until the casserole is heated through and the flavors are well combined.

9. Serve hot, garnished with additional lemon slices and parsley if desired.

Nutritional Information: Calories: 360, Protein: 32g, Carbohydrates: 22g, Fat: 14g, Fiber: 5g, Cholesterol: 80mg, Sodium: 620mg

 PRO TIP:

Add these cooking spices to aid digestion:

1. Ginger: *to reduce nausea, gas, and bloating, and relieve irritation in the digestive tract.*
2. Mint: *to decrease spasms in the gut, stomach upset and nausea, but reflux can be one of its side effects. If you get heartburn often, stick to using other herbs most of the time.*
4. Cinnamon: *to both keep blood sugar levels steady and support good digestion.*
5. Turmeric: *to reduce inflammation, relieve excess gas, abdominal pain, and bloating.*

Spicy Peanut Butter Chicken Lettuce Wraps

Ingredients

- 1 lb boneless, skinless chicken breasts, diced
- 2 tbsp olive oil
- 2 cloves garlic, minced
- 1 tbsp grated fresh ginger
- 1/4 cup soy sauce or tamari
- 2 tbsp peanut butter
- 1 tbsp honey or maple syrup
- 1 tbsp rice vinegar
- 1 tsp sriracha sauce
- 1 head butter lettuce, leaves separated
- 1 cup shredded cabbage
- 1 carrot, julienned
- 2 green onions, thinly sliced
- 1/4 cup chopped cilantro
- 1/4 cup chopped peanuts

 Prep Time: 15 min

 Cook Time: 15 min

 Serves: 4

Directions

1. Heat 1 tablespoon of olive oil in a large skillet over medium-high heat. Add the diced chicken and cook until browned and cooked through, about 5-7 minutes. Remove chicken from skillet and set aside.

2. In the same skillet, heat the remaining tablespoon of olive oil. Add the minced garlic and grated ginger, and sauté for 1-2 minutes until fragrant.

3. In a small bowl, whisk together the soy sauce, peanut butter, honey or maple syrup, rice vinegar, and sriracha sauce until smooth. Pour the sauce into the skillet with the garlic and ginger, and stir to combine.

4. Return the cooked chicken to the skillet and toss to coat in the sauce. Cook for an additional 2-3 minutes until heated through and sauce has thickened.

5. In a separate bowl, combine the shredded cabbage, julienned carrot, sliced green onions, and chopped cilantro to make the slaw.

6. To serve, spoon the spicy peanut chicken mixture onto individual lettuce leaves. Top with a generous helping of cabbage slaw and garnish with chopped peanuts. Serve with lime wedges on the side.

Nutritional Information: Calories: 320, Protein: 28g, Carbohydrates: 14g, Fat: 18g, Fiber: 4g, Cholesterol: 60mg, Sodium: 580mg

Jerk Chicken Drumsticks with Pineapple Salsa

Ingredients

- 8 chicken drumsticks
- 2 tbsp jerk seasoning
- 1/4 cup olive oil
- 2 cups diced pineapple
- 1/4 cup chopped cilantro
- 1/4 cup red onion, finely chopped
- 1 lime
- 1 tbsp of honey
- Salt and pepper to taste

 Prep Time: 10 min

 Cook Time: 30 min

 Serves: 4

Directions

1. Preheat the oven to 400°F (200°C). Line a baking sheet with parchment paper.

2. In a bowl, toss the chicken drumsticks with the jerk seasoning and olive oil until evenly coated. Season with salt and pepper.

3. Place the seasoned drumsticks on the prepared baking sheet and bake for 20-25 minutes, or until the chicken is cooked through and golden brown.

4. In a bowl, combine chopped cilantro, zest and juice of 1 lime. Whisk in all of the honey and olive oil; season to taste with salt and pepper. Stir in chopped cilantro, diced pineapple, and red onion. Season with salt and pepper.

5. Serve the jerk chicken drumsticks hot, topped with the pineapple salsa.

Nutritional Information: Calories: 320, Protein: 18g, Carbohydrates: 16g, Fat: 16g, Fiber: 0g, Cholesterol: 135mg, Sodium: 280mg

Balsamic Glazed Chicken Thighs with Brussels Sprouts

Ingredients

- 4 bone-in, skin-on chicken thighs
- 2 cups Brussels sprouts, trimmed and halved
- 2 tbsp olive oil
- 3 tbsp balsamic vinegar
- 2 tbsp honey or maple syrup
- 2 cloves garlic, minced
- 1 tsp dried thyme
- Salt and pepper, to taste
- Fresh chopped parsley for garnish (optional)

Prep Time: 10 min

Cook Time: 25 min

Serves: 4

Directions

1. Preheat the oven to 400°F (200°C). Line a baking sheet with parchment paper.

2. In a small bowl, whisk together the balsamic vinegar, honey or maple syrup, minced garlic, dried thyme, salt, and pepper.

3. Place the chicken thighs and Brussels sprouts on the prepared baking sheet. Drizzle the olive oil over the Brussels sprouts and season everything with salt and pepper.

4. Brush the balsamic glaze over the chicken thighs, ensuring they are evenly coated.

5. Roast in the preheated oven for 20-25 minutes, or until the chicken is cooked through and the Brussels sprouts are tender and caramelized.

Nutritional Information: Calories: 320, Protein: 20g, Carbohydrates: 15g, Fat: 18g, Fiber: 4g, Cholesterol: 85mg, Sodium: 260mg

Honey Mustard Drumsticks

Ingredients

- 8 chicken drumsticks
- 1/4 cup honey
- 2 tbsp Dijon mustard
- 2 tbsp apple cider vinegar
- 1 tbsp olive oil
- 2 cloves garlic, minced
- Salt and pepper to taste
- Fresh chopped parsley for garnish (optional)

Prep Time: 10 min

Cook Time: 30 min

Serves: 4

Directions

1. Preheat the oven to 400°F (200°C). Line a baking sheet with parchment paper or lightly grease with oil.

2. In a small bowl, whisk together the honey, Dijon mustard, apple cider vinegar, olive oil, minced garlic, salt, and pepper to make the glaze.

3. Place the chicken drumsticks on the prepared baking sheet. Brush each drumstick generously with the honey mustard glaze, reserving some for basting during cooking.

4. Bake the chicken drumsticks in the preheated oven for 25-30 minutes, or until they are golden brown and cooked through, flipping and basting with the remaining glaze halfway through cooking.

5. Once cooked, remove the chicken drumsticks from the oven and let them rest for a few minutes. Garnish with fresh chopped parsley if desired before serving.

Nutritional Information: Calories: 320, Protein: 18g, Carbohydrates: 16g, Fat: 16g, Fiber: 0g, Cholesterol: 135mg, Sodium: 280mg

Chapter 8: Meats

Bison Burger with Sweet Potato Fries

Prep Time: 15 min   Cook Time: 25 min   Serves: 4

Ingredients

- 1 lb ground bison
- 4 whole grain burger buns
- 2 medium sweet potatoes, cut into fries
- 2 tbsp olive oil
- 1 tsp cumin powder
- 1 tsp paprika
- Salt and pepper to taste
- 1 lime, cut into wedges
- Fresh cilantro leaves for garnish

Directions

1. Preheat the oven to 425°F (220°C) and line a baking sheet with parchment paper.
2. In a large bowl, mix the ground bison with salt and pepper to taste. Divide into 4 equal portions and shape into burger patties.
3. Place the sweet potato fries on the prepared baking sheet. Drizzle with olive oil and sprinkle with cumin, paprika, salt, and pepper. Toss to coat evenly.
4. Arrange the burger patties on the baking sheet alongside the sweet potato fries.
5. Bake in the preheated oven for 20-25 minutes, flipping the burger patties halfway through, until the burgers are cooked to your desired level of doneness and the sweet potato fries are crispy and golden brown.
6. Serve the bison burgers on whole grain buns with lime wedges on the side for squeezing over the burgers. Garnish with fresh cilantro leaves. Enjoy with the sweet potato fries.

Nutritional Information: Calories: 400, Protein: 25g, Carbohydrates: 30g, Fat: 20g, Fiber: 5g, Cholesterol: 80mg, Sodium: 450mg

Lamb Chops with Rosemary Mint Pesto

Prep Time: 10 min   Cook Time: 15 min   Serves: 4

Ingredients

- 8 lamb chops
- 2 tbsp extra virgin olive oil
- 2 cloves garlic, minced
- 2 tbsp chopped fresh rosemary
- 1 cup fresh mint leaves
- 1/4 cup pine nuts
- 1/4 cup grated Parmesan cheese
- Juice of 1 lemon
- 1/4 cup extra virgin olive oil
- Salt and pepper to taste

Directions

1. Preheat your grill or grill pan to medium-high heat.
2. Season the lamb chops generously with salt and pepper on both sides.
3. In a small bowl, mix together the olive oil, minced garlic, and chopped rosemary. Brush the mixture onto both sides of the lamb chops.
4. Place the lamb chops on the grill and cook for 5-7 minutes per side, or until they reach your desired level of doneness.
5. While the lamb chops are cooking, make the mint pesto. In a food processor, combine the mint leaves, pine nuts, Parmesan cheese, lemon juice, and extra virgin olive oil. Pulse until smooth. Season with salt and pepper to taste.
6. Once the lamb chops are done, remove them from the grill and let them rest for a few minutes before serving
7. Serve the lamb chops with pesto on top.

Nutritional Information: Calories: 420, Protein: 28g, Carbohydrates: 2g, Fat: 33g, Fiber: 1g, Cholesterol: 90mg, Sodium: 140mg

Stuffed Cabbage Rolls with Ground Beef

Prep Time: 25 min   Cook Time: 45 min   Serves: 4

Ingredients

- 1 large head of cabbage
- 1 pound lean ground beef (grass-fed preferred)
- 1/2 cup uncooked rice (brown or white)
- 1 onion, finely chopped
- 2 cloves garlic, minced
- 1 can (15 oz) tomato sauce
- 1 can (14.5 oz) diced tomatoes
- 1 tsp dried oregano
- 1 tsp dried basil
- Salt and pepper to taste
- Grated Parmesan cheese (optional)

Directions

1. Preheat your oven to 350°F (175°C). Bring a large pot of water to a boil.

2. Remove the core from the cabbage head and submerge the whole head in the boiling water. Cook for about 5 minutes, or until the outer leaves are soft and pliable. Remove from the water and set aside to cool.

3. In a mixing bowl, combine the ground beef, uncooked rice, chopped onion, minced garlic, dried oregano, dried basil, salt, and pepper. Mix until well combined.

4. Once the cabbage is cool enough to handle, carefully peel off individual leaves, being careful not to tear them. Place about 1/4 cup of the beef and rice mixture onto each cabbage leaf, then roll them up, tucking in the sides as you go. Place the cabbage rolls seam side down in a baking dish.

5. In a separate bowl, mix together the tomato sauce and diced tomatoes. Pour the tomato mixture over the cabbage rolls in the baking dish.

6. Cover the baking dish with aluminum foil and bake in the preheated oven for 40-45 minutes, or until the cabbage rolls are cooked through and rice is tender.

7. Serve the stuffed cabbage rolls hot, optionally sprinkled with grated Parmesan cheese.

Nutritional Information: Calories: 320, Protein: 22g, Carbohydrates: 25g, Fat: 14g, Fiber: 4g, Cholesterol: 60mg, Sodium: 700mg

Beef and Spinach Gluten-Free Lasagna

Prep Time: 30 min   Cook Time: 45 min   Serves: 6

Ingredients

- 1 pound gluten-free lasagna noodles
- 2 tbsp extra virgin olive oil
- 1 onion, chopped
- 2 cloves garlic, minced
- 1 pound ground beef
- 1/2 tsp turmeric powder
- 1/2 tsp black pepper
- 2 cups tomato sauce
- 1 cup ricotta cheese (or a non-dairy alternative like almond ricotta)
- 1 egg, beaten
- 2 cups fresh spinach, chopped
- 2 cups shredded mozzarella cheese

Directions

1. Cook the gluten-free lasagna noodles according to package instructions; drain and set aside.

2. In a skillet, heat the olive oil over medium heat. Add onion and garlic, sauté until soft. Add ground beef, turmeric, and black pepper, and cook until browned. Stir in the tomato sauce.

3. In a bowl, mix ricotta cheese with the beaten egg and spinach.

4. In a baking dish, layer noodles, beef sauce, ricotta mixture, and mozzarella. Repeat layers, finishing with mozzarella on top.

5. Bake at 375°F (190°C) for 25 minutes or until bubbly and golden on top.

Nutritional Information: Calories: 400, Protein: 30g, Carbohydrates: 34g, Fat: 20g, Fiber: 5g, Cholesterol: 80mg, Sodium: 340mg

Spiced Lamb with Veggies and Raisins

Prep Time: 25 min   Cook Time: 2 hours   Serves: 4

Ingredients

- 1 pound lamb shoulder, cut into chunks
- 2 large sweet potatoes, peeled and cubed
- 2 tbsp extra virgin olive oil
- 1 onion, chopped
- 2 cloves garlic, minced
- 1 tsp turmeric powder
- 1 tsp cumin powder
- 1/2 tsp cinnamon powder
- 1/4 tsp ground ginger
- 1/2 tsp paprika powder
- 1/2 cup golden raisins (sulfur-free)
- 2 cups vegetable broth
- 2 carrots, peeled and sliced
- 1 zucchini, sliced
- Salt and pepper
- Fresh cilantro, chopped for garnish

Directions

1. In a tagine or heavy pot, heat the olive oil over medium heat. Add the lamb and brown on all sides, then remove and set aside.
2. In the same pot sauté the onion and garlic until soft.
3. Add turmeric, cumin, cinnamon, ginger, and paprika, cooking for 1 minute until fragrant.
4. Return the lamb to the pot. Add vegetable broth, golden raisins, sweet potatoes, carrots and zucchini. Bring to a simmer. Season with salt and pepper to taste.
5. Cover with the lid and let it cook on low heat for about 1.5 to 2 hours, or until the lamb is tender and the flavors are well blended.
6. Garnish with fresh cilantro before serving and serve over quinoa or rice.

Nutritional Information: Calories: 495, Protein: 38g, Carbohydrates: 52g, Fat: 18g, Fiber: 7g, Cholesterol: 90mg, Sodium: 420mg

Ground Beef Stuffed Portobello Mushrooms

Prep Time: 20 min   Cook Time: 25 min   Serves: 4

Ingredients

- 4 large portobello mushroom caps, stems removed
- 1 tbsp extra virgin olive oil
- 1/2 red onion, finely chopped
- 2 cloves garlic, minced
- 1 pound ground lean beef (grass-fed preferred)
- 1/2 tsp turmeric powder
- 1/2 tsp sea salt
- 1/4 tsp freshly ground black pepper
- 1/2 cup crumbled feta cheese
- 1/4 cup fresh parsley, chopped
- 1 tbsp apple cider vinegar

Directions

1. Preheat the oven to 375°F (190°C). Brush the mushrooms with olive oil and place them gill-side up on a baking sheet.
2. Heat a skillet over medium heat, add the onion and garlic, and sauté until translucent. Add the ground beef, turmeric, salt, pepper, and apple cider vinegar. Cook until the beef is fully cooked.
3. Spoon the beef mixture into the mushroom caps and top with feta cheese if using.
4. Bake in the preheated oven for 20 minutes, or until the mushrooms are tender.
5. Garnish with fresh parsley before serving.

Nutritional Information: Calories: 270, Protein: 28g, Carbohydrates: 10g, Fat: 15g, Fiber: 3g, Cholesterol: 65mg, Sodium: 320mg

Venison Backstrap with Blackberry Sage Sauce

Prep Time: 20 min   Cook Time: 30 min   Serves: 4

Ingredients

- 2 lbs venison backstrap, trimmed
- 1 tbsp extra virgin olive oil
- Salt and freshly ground black pepper to taste
- 1 cup fresh blackberries
- 1/4 cup balsamic vinegar
- 1/4 cup pomegranate juice
- 2 tbsp honey
- 2 tbsp fresh sage, finely chopped
- 2 cloves garlic, minced
- 1/4 tsp cinnamon powder
- 1 tbsp ground flaxseed

Directions

1. Preheat a skillet over medium-high heat and add the extra virgin olive oil. Season the venison backstrap with salt, black pepper, and cinnamon. Sear the venison in the hot skillet for about 5 minutes on each side or until it reaches your desired level of doneness. Remove the venison from the skillet and let it rest.

2. In the same skillet, add the blackberries, balsamic vinegar, pomegranate juice, honey, sage, and minced garlic. Cook over medium heat, stirring and mashing the blackberries until the sauce has reduced and thickened, about 15-20 minutes.

3. Stir in the ground flaxseed into the sauce for the last few minutes of cooking to incorporate well and thicken the sauce slightly.

4. Slice the rested venison into medallions. Serve the medallions with the blackberry sage sauce spooned over the top.

Nutritional Information: Calories: 340, Protein: 36g, Carbohydrates: 18g, Fat: 13g, Fiber: 4g, Cholesterol: 90mg, Sodium: 75mg

---

Beef Fajita Bowls with Wild Rice

Prep Time: 20 min   Cook Time: 50 min   Serves: 4

Ingredients

- 1 lb beef sirloin, thinly sliced
- 2 cups cooked wild rice
- 1 tbsp extra virgin olive oil
- 1 large red bell pepper, sliced
- 1 large yellow bell pepper, sliced
- 1 medium onion, sliced
- 1 tsp turmeric powder
- 1 tsp smoked paprika
- 1/2 tsp garlic powder
- 1/4 tsp ground black pepper
- 1/4 tsp cayenne pepper
- 1 tbsp apple cider vinegar
- 1/2 cup fresh parsley, chopped
- 1 avocado, sliced
- 2 tbsp pumpkin seeds
- Lime wedges

Directions

1. Cook the wild rice according to package instructions. Set aside.

2. Marinate the thinly sliced beef in apple cider vinegar for at least 10 minutes before cooking.

3. Heat the extra virgin olive oil in a large skillet over medium-high heat. Add the marinated beef and cook for about 5-6 minutes, or until browned.

4. Add the bell peppers, and onion to the skillet. Sprinkle with turmeric, smoked paprika, garlic powder, black pepper, and cayenne pepper. Stir well to coat and cook for another 5-7 minutes, until the vegetables are soft and the beef is fully cooked.

5. To assemble, divide the wild rice among bowls. Top with the beef and vegetable mixture. Add sliced avocado and sprinkle with pumpkin seeds. Garnish with fresh parsley and lime wedges.

Nutritional Information: Calories: 330, Protein: 27g, Carbohydrates: 32g, Fat: 19g, Fiber: 7g, Cholesterol: 64mg, Sodium: 130mg

Beef Meatballs with Mint Tomato Sauce

Prep Time: 15 min   Cook Time: 35 min   Serves: 4

Ingredients

- 1 lb ground beef (grass-fed preferred)
- 1 egg
- 1/3 cup finely chopped fresh mint
- 1/3 cup of finely chopped flat leaf parsley
- 3 cloves garlic, minced
- 1 tbsp ground flaxseed
- 1 tsp dried oregano
- 1/2 tsp turmeric powder
- Salt and freshly ground black pepper

For Tomato Sauce:
- 1 can (14.5 oz) diced tomatoes
- 2 cloves of garlic, minced
- 2 sprigs of thyme
- 1/2 tsp of red pepper flakes
- Salt and pepper
- 4 tbsp of olive oil
- 1 cup chopped kale
- A splash of lemon juice

Directions

1. Preheat the oven to 375°F.
2. In a large bowl, mix together the ground beef, egg, mint, garlic, flaxseed, oregano, turmeric, salt, and pepper until well combined.
3. Form the mixture into meatballs and place on a baking sheet lined with parchment paper.
4. Bake the meatballs for 25 minutes or until cooked through.
5. While the meatballs are baking, in a saucepan, add the garlic, pepper flakes, and thyme and sauté for about a minute (until the garlic becomes fragrant). Stir in the diced tomatoes in their juice and lower the heat to medium. Add chopped kale and simmer for about 10-15 minutes.
6. Add a splash of lemon juice, and season with salt and pepper to taste and chopped mint.
7. Add the cooked meatballs to the pot with the sauce and toss gently to coat them.

Nutritional Information: Calories: 350, Protein: 24g, Carbohydrates: 15g, Fat: 22g, Fiber: 3g, Cholesterol: 120mg, Sodium: 350mg

Rustic Beef Tacos with Black Beans

Prep Time: 35 min   Cook Time: 15 min   Serves: 4

Ingredients

- 1 lb roasted beef (grass-fed preferred), sliced thinly
- 1 cup black beans, cooked
- 1 red onion, thinly sliced
- 1 red bell pepper, thinly sliced
- Organic corn or almond flour tortillas
- 1/2 tsp turmeric powder
- 1 tsp cumin powder
- 1 tsp coriander powder
- 1 tbsp extra virgin olive oil
- 2 cloves garlic, minced
- 1/2 cup kale, finely chopped
- 1/4 cup diced tomatoes
- 1/4 cup feta cheese, crumbled (optional)
- 1 tbsp tahini
- Fresh parsley, chopped
- Fresh lemon juice

Directions

1. Heat the olive oil in a skillet over medium heat; add garlic and sauté until fragrant, about 1-2 minutes.
2. Add the beef to the skillet; season with turmeric, cumin, and coriander. Cook until browned, about 5-6 minutes.
3. Mix in the red onion and bell pepper, cooking until softened, about 5 minutes.
4. Stir in the black beans and kale, cooking until the kale is wilted and the beans are heated through, about 2-3 minutes.
5. Warm the tortillas in a separate pan over medium heat for about 30 seconds each side, then fill with the beef mixture, top with tomatoes, feta cheese, and a drizzle of tahini. Garnish with parsley and a squeeze of lemon juice.

Nutritional Information: Calories: 380, Protein: 26g, Carbohydrates: 24g, Fat: 20g, Fiber: 5g, Cholesterol: 60mg, Sodium: 320mg

Golden Spice Lamb Meatballs with Zoodles

Ingredients

For Lamb Meatballs:

- 1 lb ground lamb (grass-fed preferred)
- 1/4 cup almond flour
- 1 large egg, beaten
- 3 cloves garlic, minced
- 1 tsp cumin powder
- 1 tsp coriander
- 1 tsp turmeric powder
- 1/2 tsp salt
- 1/4 tsp black pepper
- 2 tbsp coconut oil

For Yogurt Sauce:

- 1 cup Greek yogurt
- 1 cucumber, seeded and finely grated
- 2 cloves garlic, minced
- 1 tbsp lemon juice
- 1 tbsp fresh dill, chopped
- Salt and pepper to taste

For the Zucchini Noodles:

- 4 large zucchini, spiralized
- 1 tbsp olive oil

Prep Time: 30 min   Cook Time: 20 min   Serves: 4

Directions

1. Prepare the Meatballs: In a mixing bowl, combine the ground lamb, almond flour, egg, garlic, cumin, coriander, turmeric, salt, and pepper. Mix thoroughly until the ingredients are well integrated. Form the mixture into 1-inch meatballs.

2. Heat coconut oil in a skillet over medium heat. Add the meatballs and cook, turning occasionally, until they are evenly browned and fully cooked, about 10-12 minutes. Remove from the skillet and keep warm.

3. In a separate bowl, mix the Greek yogurt, grated cucumber, garlic, lemon juice, and dill. Season with salt and pepper to taste, ensuring all components are well combined.

4. Warm olive oil in a large non-stick skillet over medium heat. Add the zucchini noodles and sauté for about 2-3 minutes until just tender, maintaining a bit of crunch.

5. Distribute the zucchini noodles evenly among plates. Top with lamb meatballs and a generous dollop of yogurt sauce.

Nutritional Information: Calories: 495, Protein: 30g, Carbohydrates: 20g, Fat: 35g, Fiber: 5g, Cholesterol: 105mg, Sodium: 600mg

 PRO TIP:

Anti-Inflammatory Veggie Noodles Ideas to Substitute for Pasta or Rice:

Zucchini Noodles, Carrot Noodles, Sweet Potato Noodles, Squash Noodles, Broccoli Stem Noodles, Parsnip Noodles, Turnip Noodles, Spaghetti Squash, Shaved Asparagus, and Shredded Brussels Sprouts!

Savory Wine-Braised Beef with Veggies

Prep Time: 20 min   Cook Time: 2 hours   Serves: 4

Ingredients

- 1.5 lbs beef chuck, cut into cubes
- 2 tbsp extra virgin olive oil
- 1 large onion, chopped
- 3 carrots, sliced
- 3 cloves garlic, minced
- 2 cups mushrooms, preferably shiitake
- 1 bottle (750 ml) dry red wine, organic if possible
- 2 cups low-sodium beef broth
- 1 tbsp tomato paste

- 1 tsp dried thyme
- 2 bay leaves
- 1/2 tsp turmeric powder
- 1/2 tsp ground ginger
- Fresh parsley, chopped
- 2 tbsp fresh lemon juice
- Salt and black pepper to taste
- 1 tbsp ground flaxseed (optional)

Directions

1. Heat the extra virgin olive oil in a large pot over medium-high heat. Add the beef cubes and sear until browned on all sides, about 5-7 minutes. Remove the beef and set aside.

2. In the same pot, add the onion and carrots. Cook until the onion becomes translucent and carrots start to soften, about 5 minutes.

3. Stir in the garlic, mushrooms, turmeric, and ground ginger. Cook for another 3 minutes until the mushrooms begin to brown and the spices are fragrant.

4. Return the beef to the pot. Add the red wine, beef broth, tomato paste, thyme, and bay leaves. Bring to a boil, then reduce the heat to low and let simmer covered for about 1 to 1.5 hours, or until the beef is tender.

5. Stir in the fresh lemon juice and optional ground flaxseed during the last 5 minutes of cooking. Season with salt and black pepper to taste. Garnish with fresh parsley before serving.

Nutritional Information: Calories: 420, Protein: 36g, Carbohydrates: 18g, Fat: 18g, Fiber: 5g, Cholesterol: 90mg, Sodium: 350mg

Beef and Sweet Potato Hash

Prep Time: 25 min   Cook Time: 15 min   Serves: 4

Ingredients

- 1 lb ground beef (grass-fed preferred)
- 2 large sweet potatoes, peeled and diced
- 1 large onion, diced
- 1 red bell pepper, diced
- 2 cloves garlic, minced
- 1 tsp smoked paprika
- 1 tsp cumin powder
- 1 tsp dried thyme

- Salt and pepper to taste
- 2 tbsp olive oil
- 2 green onions, sliced (for garnish)
- 1 avocado, diced (optional, for garnish)
- Hot sauce (optional, for serving)

Directions

1. Heat 1 tablespoon of olive oil in a large skillet over medium heat. Add the ground beef, breaking it apart with a spoon, and cook until browned. Remove beef from the skillet and set aside.

2. In the same skillet, add the remaining tablespoon of olive oil. Add the diced sweet potatoes and cook for about 10 minutes, stirring occasionally, until they begin to soften.

3. Add the diced onion, red bell pepper, and garlic to the skillet. Cook for an additional 5 minutes, or until the vegetables are tender.

4. Return the cooked ground beef to the skillet. Stir in the smoked paprika, cumin, dried thyme, salt, and pepper. Cook for another 5 minutes, allowing the flavors to meld together. Garnish with sliced green onions and diced avocado, if using. Serve with hot sauce if desired.

Nutritional Information: Calories: 450, Protein: 25g, Carbohydrates: 30g, Fat: 25g, Fiber: 6g, Cholesterol: 70mg, Sodium: 450mg

Delectable Coconut Lamb Curry

Ingredients

- 1 lb lamb, cut into cubes
- 1 tbsp extra virgin olive oil
- 1 large onion, diced
- 2 cloves garlic, minced
- 2 tbsp fresh ginger, grated
- 1 tbsp turmeric powder
- 1 tsp cumin powder
- 1 tsp coriander powder
- 1/2 tsp black pepper
- 1/2 tsp cinnamon powder
- 1/4 tsp cayenne pepper (optional)
- 1 can (14 oz) diced tomatoes
- 1 can (14 oz) coconut milk
- 1 cup chopped carrots
- 1 cup chopped sweet potatoes
- 1 cup broccoli florets
- 1/2 cup chopped kale
- Salt to taste
- Fresh cilantro, chopped (for garnish)
- 1 tbsp apple cider vinegar
- 2 tbsp flaxseed meal

Prep Time: 20 min

Cook Time: 1 hour

Serves: 4

Directions

1. Heat the extra virgin olive oil in a large pot over medium heat. Add the onion, garlic, and ginger, cooking until the onion becomes translucent.

2. Mix in the turmeric, cumin, coriander, black pepper, cinnamon, and cayenne pepper. Cook for about 2 minutes until fragrant, stirring frequently.

3. Add the lamb cubes to the pot and brown them on all sides.

4. Pour in the diced tomatoes, coconut milk, and apple cider vinegar. Bring the mixture to a simmer, then reduce the heat to low.

5. Stir in the carrots and sweet potatoes. Cover and let it simmer for about 40 minutes.

6. Add the broccoli and kale to the pot, and continue to simmer for an additional 10 minutes, or until the vegetables are tender and the lamb is fully cooked.

7. Stir in the flaxseed meal and cook for another 5 minutes to thicken the sauce slightly.

8. Season with salt to taste. Garnish with fresh cilantro before serving.

Nutritional Information: Calories: 510, Protein: 26g, Carbohydrates: 38g, Fat: 30g, Fiber: 9g, Cholesterol: 80mg, Sodium: 130mg

 PRO TIP:

Turmeric: *Adding turmeric not only boosts the anti-inflammatory properties but also gives the dish a warm, earthy flavor. Combine it with a pinch of black pepper, healthy fats like a nut butters, avocado or olive oil and use with heat to enhance absorption up to 12 times.*

Garlic: *Fresh garlic is a powerhouse for fighting inflammation. Its active compound, allicin, has been shown to reduce inflammation and boost immune function. For maximum allicin that will also help it stay intact during cooking, crush, chop or mince garlic and keep it away from heat for 10 minutes.*

Zesty Beef and Broccoli Casserole

Prep Time: 20 min   Cook Time: 35 min   Serves: 4

Ingredients

- 1 lb lean ground beef (grass-fed preferred)
- 3 cups broccoli florets, fresh or frozen
- 1 large onion, diced
- 3 cloves garlic, minced
- 1 cup mushrooms, sliced
- 1 tbsp extra virgin olive oil
- 1 tbsp grated ginger
- 1/2 tsp turmeric powder
- 1/2 tsp ground black pepper
- 1/2 tsp sea salt
- 1 cup bone broth
- 2 tbsp arrowroot powder (or 1 tbsp of rice flour)
- 1/2 cup coconut cream
- 1/4 cup grated parmesan cheese
- 1/3 cup ground flaxseed
- 1/4 cup chopped parsley

Directions

1. Preheat your oven to 375°F (190°C). Heat the olive oil in a large skillet over medium heat. Add the garlic, onion, and ginger, and sauté until the onion is translucent and fragrant, about 6-7 minutes.

2. Increase the heat to medium-high and add the ground beef to the skillet. Cook until browned, breaking it apart as it cooks, about 10 minutes.

3. Stir in the broccoli and mushrooms, and cook for an additional 5 minutes. Season with turmeric, black pepper, and sea salt.

4. In a small bowl, mix the arrowroot powder or rice flour with a little cold bone broth until smooth. Pour this mixture and the remaining bone broth into the skillet. Bring to a simmer, stirring continuously, until the mixture thickens, then mix in the coconut cream.

5. Transfer the beef and vegetable mixture to a baking dish. Combine with bone broth & coconut cream mixture and the ground flaxseed. Sprinkle parmesan cheese on top. Bake in the preheated oven for 20 minutes, or until the topping is golden brown. Garnish with chopped parsley before serving.

Nutritional Information: Calories: 390, Protein: 30g, Carbohydrates: 16g, Fat: 24g, Fiber: 6g, Cholesterol: 70mg, Sodium: 280mg

Herbed Butter Prime Rib Roast with Broccoli

Prep Time: 20 min   Cook Time: 1.5 hours   Serves: 4

Ingredients

- 1 (4-pound) prime rib roast
- 1/2 cup unsalted butter, softened
- 4 cloves garlic, minced
- 1 tbsp fresh rosemary, chopped
- 1 tbsp fresh thyme, chopped
- 1 tbsp fresh parsley, chopped
- 2 tsp salt
- 1 tsp black pepper
- 1 lb broccoli florets
- 2 tbsp olive oil
- 1 tsp garlic powder
- Salt and pepper

Directions

1. Preheat your oven to 450°F (232°C). In a small bowl, combine the butter, garlic, rosemary, thyme, parsley, salt, and black pepper. Mix until well combined. Rub the herbed butter mixture all over the prime rib roast.

2. Place the roast on a rack in a roasting pan, fat side up. Roast in the preheated oven for 15 minutes. Reduce the oven temperature to 325°F (163°C) and continue roasting until the internal temperature reaches 120°F (49°C) for medium-rare, about 1 hour and 15 minutes.

3. While the roast is cooking, toss the broccoli florets with olive oil, garlic powder, salt, and pepper. Spread the broccoli on a baking sheet.

4. When the roast has about 25 minutes left, place the broccoli in the oven. Roast until tender and slightly crispy, about 20-25 minutes. Remove the roast from the oven and let it rest for 15 minutes before slicing. Serve with roasted broccoli.

Nutritional Information: Calories: 850, Protein: 50g, Carbohydrates: 10g, Fat: 70g, Fiber: 4g, Cholesterol: 220mg, Sodium: 800mg

Fiery Beef and Cauli-Veggie Plate

 Prep Time: 15 min   Cook Time: 15 min   Serves: 4

Ingredients

- 1 lb ground beef (grass-fed preferred)
- 1 head cauliflower, riced
- 2 tbsp sesame oil
- 3 cloves garlic, minced
- 1 small onion, diced
- 1/4 cup soy sauce (or tamari for gluten-free)
- 2 tbsp pure maple syrup
- 1 tbsp grated ginger
- 1 tbsp sriracha
- 1 cup shredded carrots
- 1 cup chopped bell pepper
- 1/2 cup sliced green onions
- 1 tbsp sesame seeds
- Salt and pepper

Directions

1. Heat 1 tablespoon of sesame oil in a large skillet over medium heat. Add the minced garlic and diced onion, sauté until fragrant, about 2-3 minutes.

2. Add the ground beef to the skillet, breaking it apart with a spatula. Cook until browned, about 5-7 minutes. Drain excess fat if necessary.

3. Stir in soy sauce, pure maple syrup, grated ginger, and sriracha. Cook for another 2-3 minutes until the sauce is well combined and heated through. Add shredded carrots and bell pepper, cooking for another 2 minutes.

4. In a separate skillet, heat the remaining sesame oil over medium heat. Add the riced cauliflower and cook, stirring frequently, until tender, about 5 minutes. Season with salt and pepper.

5. Serve the beef over the cauliflower rice, garnishing with sliced green onions and sesame seeds.

Nutritional Information: Calories: 315, Protein: 25g, Carbohydrates: 17g, Fat: 18g, Fiber: 4g, Cholesterol: 70mg, Sodium: 720mg

Lemon Veal Chops with Wild Rice

 Prep Time: 20 min   Cook Time: 40 min   Serves: 4

Ingredients

- 4 veal chops (about 1 inch thick)
- 2 tbsp extra virgin olive oil
- Salt and pepper to taste
- 1 cup wild rice
- 2 cups water or low-sodium vegetable broth
- 1 tsp turmeric powder
- 1 tsp ground ginger
- 1 lemon, zested and juiced
- 2 garlic cloves, minced
- 1/4 cup fresh parsley, finely chopped
- 1/4 cup fresh basil, finely chopped
- 1/4 cup fresh mint, finely chopped
- 1 tbsp capers, drained and chopped (optional)

Directions

1. In a small saucepan, bring 2 cups of water or low-sodium vegetable broth to a boil. Add wild rice, ground turmeric, and ground ginger. Reduce heat to low, cover, and simmer for 40 minutes or until tender. Fluff with a fork and set aside.

2. Preheat your oven to 375°F (190°C). Rub the veal chops with olive oil and season generously with salt and pepper. Place the chops on a baking sheet and bake for 20-25 minutes, or until they reach an internal temperature of 145°F (medium-rare) to 160°F (medium).

3. While the veal chops are baking combine lemon zest, lemon juice, minced garlic, parsley, basil, mint, and capers in a small bowl. Mix well and set aside.

4. Once the veal chops are done, let them rest for a few minutes. Serve the chops topped with the lemon mixture, accompanied by a side of wild rice.

Nutritional Information: Calories: 450, Protein: 35g, Carbohydrates: 30g, Fat: 20g, Fiber: 4g, Cholesterol: 100mg, Sodium: 150mg

Venison Steak with Cranberry Sauce and Root Vegetables

Ingredients

For Venison Steak:

- 4 venison steaks (about 6 oz each)
- Salt and pepper to taste
- 2 tbsp extra virgin olive oil
- 2 garlic cloves, minced
- 1 tsp fresh thyme, chopped

For Cranberry Sauce:

- 1 cup fresh cranberries
- 1/2 cup orange juice
- 1/4 cup honey
- 1/4 tsp cinnamon powder

For Roasted Root Vegetables:

- 2 large carrots, peeled and chopped
- 2 parsnips, peeled and chopped
- 1 sweet potato, peeled and chopped
- 1 red onion, peeled and quartered
- 2 tbsp extra virgin olive oil
- Salt and pepper to taste
- 1 tsp fresh rosemary, chopped

 Prep Time: 20 min

 Cook Time: 40 min

 Serves: 4

Directions

1. Preheat the oven to 400°F (200°C). In a large bowl, toss the carrots, parsnips, sweet potato, and red onion with olive oil, salt, pepper, and rosemary. Spread the vegetables on a baking sheet and roast for 35-40 minutes, or until tender and golden brown, stirring halfway through.

2. While the vegetables are roasting, prepare the cranberry sauce. In a small saucepan, combine the cranberries, orange juice, honey, and cinnamon. Bring to a boil over medium heat, then reduce the heat and simmer for 10-15 minutes, or until the cranberries have burst and the sauce has thickened.

3. Season the venison steaks with salt, pepper, minced garlic, and fresh thyme. Heat olive oil in a large skillet over medium-high heat. Add the steaks and cook for 4-5 minutes per side for medium-rare, or until they reach your desired doneness. Remove from the skillet and let rest for a few minutes.

4. Serve the venison steaks topped with cranberry sauce, alongside the roasted root vegetables.

Nutritional Information: Calories: 550, Protein: 42g, Carbohydrates: 48g, Fat: 20g, Fiber: 8g, Cholesterol: 120mg, Sodium: 500mg

 PRO TIP:

Cranberries combat oxidative stress and have major anti-inflammatory effects, thanks to their high amounts of antioxidants, especially anthocyanins and flavanols. Furthermore, they support immune function with high vitamin C, improve heart health, lower bad cholesterol (LDL) and increase good cholesterol (HDL), reduce gut inflammation, prevent Urinary Tract Infections (UTIs), promote skin health and are anti-aging!

Chapter 9: Vegetarian

Butternut Squash with Cranberries and Pecans

Prep Time: 15 min   Cook Time: 30 min   Serves: 4

Ingredients

- 1 medium butternut squash, peeled, seeded, and cubed
- 1 cup fresh cranberries
- 1/2 cup pecans, roughly chopped
- 2 tbsp extra virgin olive oil
- 2 tbsp maple syrup
- 1 tsp cinnamon powder
- 1/2 tsp nutmeg
- Salt to taste

Directions

1. Preheat the oven to 375°F (190°C). Line a baking sheet with parchment paper.

2. In a large bowl, combine the cubed butternut squash, cranberries, and pecans. Drizzle with olive oil and maple syrup, then sprinkle with cinnamon, nutmeg, and salt. Toss everything together until well coated.

3. Spread the mixture evenly on the prepared baking sheet. Roast in the preheated oven for about 25-30 minutes, or until the squash is tender and lightly caramelized, stirring halfway through the cooking time.

4. Remove from the oven and let cool slightly before serving.

Nutritional Information: Calories: 290, Protein: 3g, Carbohydrates: 33g, Fat: 18g, Fiber: 6g, Cholesterol: 0mg, Sodium: 10mg

Grilled Eggplant Steaks with Chimichurri

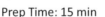

Prep Time: 15 min   Cook Time: 10 min   Serves: 4

Ingredients

- 2 large eggplants, sliced into 1/2-inch-thick rounds
- 2 tbsp extra virgin olive oil
- Salt and pepper to taste

For Chimichurri:

- 1 cup fresh parsley, finely chopped
- 1/4 cup fresh oregano leaves, finely chopped
- 3 cloves garlic, minced
- 1/2 cup extra virgin olive oil
- 2 tbsp red wine vinegar
- 1 tsp red pepper flakes
- Salt to taste

Directions

1. Preheat the grill to medium-high heat. Brush both sides of the eggplant slices with olive oil and season with salt and pepper.

2. Grill the eggplant slices for about 5 minutes on each side, until tender and grill marks appear.

3. To make the chimichurri, combine the parsley, oregano, minced garlic, olive oil, red wine vinegar, red pepper flakes, and salt in a bowl. Stir well to blend.

4. Serve the grilled eggplant steaks topped with a generous amount of chimichurri sauce.

Nutritional Information: Calories: 320, Protein: 2g, Carbohydrates: 14g, Fat: 29g, Fiber: 6g, Cholesterol: 0mg, Sodium: 40mg

Stuffed Bell Peppers with Lentils and Walnuts

Prep Time: 20 min   Cook Time: 40 min   Serves: 4

Ingredients

- 4 large bell peppers, tops cut off and seeds removed
- 1 cup cooked green lentils
- 1/2 cup walnuts, finely chopped
- 1 medium onion, finely chopped
- 2 cloves garlic, minced
- 1 carrot, grated
- 1 zucchini, grated

- 2 tbsp extra virgin olive oil
- 1 tsp dried basil
- 1 tsp dried oregano
- 1/2 tsp salt
- 1/4 tsp black pepper
- 1/2 cup tomato sauce
- 1/4 cup water
- Fresh parsley, chopped

Directions

1. Preheat the oven to 375°F (190°C). Heat olive oil in a skillet over medium heat. Sauté onion and garlic until translucent, about 5 minutes.

2. Add the grated carrot and zucchini to the skillet and cook for an additional 5 minutes. Stir in the cooked lentils, walnuts, basil, oregano, salt, and pepper, and cook for another 5 minutes until well combined.

3. Arrange the bell peppers in a baking dish. Spoon the lentil-walnut mixture into each pepper, pressing down to pack tightly. Mix the tomato sauce with water and pour into the bottom of the dish around the peppers.

4. Cover with foil and bake in the preheated oven for 30 minutes. Remove the foil and bake for an additional 10 minutes, or until the peppers are tender and the filling is heated through.

5. Garnish with fresh parsley before serving.

Nutritional Information: Calories: 290, Protein: 10g, Carbohydrates: 30g, Fat: 16g, Fiber: 9g, Cholesterol: 0mg, Sodium: 300mg

Roasted Carrot and Fennel

Prep Time: 15 min   Cook Time: 30 min   Serves: 4

Ingredients

- 6 large carrots, peeled and cut into batons
- 2 fennel bulbs, trimmed and sliced
- 2 tbsp olive oil
- Salt and black pepper to taste
- 2 tbsp tahini

- 1 lemon, juiced
- 1 garlic clove, minced
- 2 tbsp warm water
- 1 tbsp honey
- 1/4 cup chopped parsley

Directions

1. Preheat the oven to 400°F (200°C). In a large mixing bowl, toss the carrots and fennel with olive oil, salt, and pepper. Spread the vegetables on a baking sheet in a single layer.

2. Roast in the preheated oven for about 30 minutes, or until the vegetables are tender and caramelized, turning once halfway through cooking.

3. While the vegetables are roasting, prepare the tahini dressing. In a small bowl, whisk together tahini, lemon juice, minced garlic, honey, and warm water until smooth.

4. Remove the vegetables from the oven and let them cool slightly. Place the roasted carrots and fennel in a serving dish.

5. Drizzle the tahini dressing over the vegetables and sprinkle with chopped parsley before serving.

Nutritional Information: Calories: 230, Protein: 4g, Carbohydrates: 24g, Fat: 14g, Fiber: 6g, Cholesterol: 0mg, Sodium: 150mg

Grilled Polenta Cakes with Roasted Red Pepper Sauce

Ingredients

For Polenta Cakes:

- 1 cup polenta (cornmeal)
- 4 cups water
- 1 tsp salt
- 1 tbsp extra virgin olive oil

For Roasted Red Pepper Sauce:

- 2 large red bell peppers
- 1 small onion, chopped
- 2 cloves garlic, minced
- 1 tbsp olive oil
- 1/2 tsp smoked paprika
- Salt and pepper to taste
- Fresh basil leaves, for garnish

 Prep Time: 30 min

 Cook Time: 20 min

 Serves: 4

Directions

1. In a medium saucepan, bring 4 cups of water to a boil. Gradually whisk in the polenta and salt. Reduce the heat to low and continue to stir until the polenta thickens and is fully cooked, about 15-20 minutes. Once cooked, spread the polenta into a greased baking dish, forming an even layer about 1/2 inch thick. Allow to cool and set for about 30 minutes.

2. While the polenta is setting, roast the red bell peppers by placing them under a broiler or over an open flame until the skin is charred and blistered. Place the roasted peppers in a bowl and cover with plastic wrap to steam for 10 minutes. Peel away the skins, remove the seeds, and chop.

3. Heat 1 tbsp olive oil in a skillet over medium heat. Add chopped onion and minced garlic, and sauté until onion is translucent, about 5 minutes. Add the chopped roasted peppers and smoked paprika, and cook for another 5 minutes. Transfer the mixture to a blender and puree until smooth. Season with salt and pepper to taste.

4. Preheat a grill or grill pan over medium-high heat. Cut the set polenta into squares or circles and brush each side with olive oil. Grill the polenta cakes for about 3-4 minutes on each side, or until they have nice grill marks and are heated through.

5. Serve the grilled polenta cakes topped with the roasted red pepper sauce, garnished with fresh basil leaves.

Nutritional Information: Calories: 210, Protein: 4g, Carbohydrates: 32g, Fat: 7g, Fiber: 4g, Cholesterol: 0mg, Sodium: 600mg

 PRO TIP:

Polenta is a versatile dish that pairs well with various anti-inflammatory ingredients, making it perfect for both sweet and savory options. Some ideas to add to a health-boosting polenta include:
- Spinach and Kale: are packed with vitamins A, C, and K and other antioxidants.
- Powerhouse Trio of turmeric, black pepper and cinnamon such as in polenta with sauteed apples.
- Cayenne Pepper and Paprika: contain capsaicin, which has anti-inflammatory benefits.
- Garlic and Onion: are high in sulfur compounds that fight inflammation.
- Fresh Ginger: contains gingerols that provide strong anti-inflammatory effects.
- Rosemary and Thyme: are rich in rosmarinic acid and thymol, which reduce inflammation.
- Parsley and Cilantro: are high in flavonoids and antioxidants.
- Chia Seeds: are loaded with omega-3 fatty acids and fiber.

Crispy Baked Tahini Cauliflower Bites

Prep Time: 15 min   Cook Time: 25 min   Serves: 4

Ingredients

- 1 large head of cauliflower, cut into florets
- 2 tbsp extra virgin olive oil
- 1 tsp garlic powder
- 1 tsp smoked paprika
- 1/2 tsp cayenne pepper
- Salt and black pepper
- 1/4 cup tahini
- 2 tbsp lemon juice
- 1 tbsp maple syrup
- 1 clove garlic, minced
- 2-4 tbsp warm water
- Fresh parsley, chopped

Directions

1. Preheat the oven to 400°F (200°C) and line a baking sheet with parchment paper.

2. In a large bowl, toss the cauliflower florets with olive oil, garlic powder, smoked paprika, cayenne pepper, salt, and black pepper until well coated.

3. Spread the cauliflower in a single layer on the prepared baking sheet. Bake for 25 minutes, or until golden and crispy, flipping halfway through.

4. While the cauliflower is baking, prepare the tahini drizzle by whisking together tahini, lemon juice, maple syrup, minced garlic, and warm water in a small bowl until smooth.

5. Once the cauliflower is done, drizzle the tahini sauce over the hot cauliflower and sprinkle with chopped parsley.

Nutritional Information: Calories: 210, Protein: 6g, Carbohydrates: 18g, Fat: 14g, Fiber: 5g, Cholesterol: 0mg, Sodium: 65mg

Spaghetti Squash with Marinara Sauce

Prep Time: 15 min   Cook Time: 45 min   Serves: 4

Ingredients

- 1 large spaghetti squash (about 3 pounds)
- 2 tbsp extra virgin olive oil
- 1 onion, finely chopped
- 3 cloves garlic, minced
- 1 can (28 oz) crushed tomatoes
- 1 tsp turmeric powder
- 1 tsp dried basil
- 1 tsp dried oregano
- 1/2 tsp black pepper
- 1/2 tsp crushed red pepper flakes
- Salt to taste
- 1/2 cup chopped kale
- 1/4 cup fresh basil, chopped
- 2 tbsp nutritional yeast

Directions

1. Preheat the oven to 400°F (200°C). Halve the spaghetti squash lengthwise and scoop out the seeds. Drizzle the inside with 1 tablespoon of olive oil and a sprinkle of salt. Place the squash halves cut-side down on a baking sheet and roast in the oven for about 30-35 minutes, until the flesh is tender.

2. Heat the remaining tablespoon of olive oil in a saucepan over medium heat. Add the onion and garlic, sautéing until the onion is translucent, about 5-7 minutes.

3. Stir in the crushed tomatoes, turmeric, basil, oregano, black pepper, and red pepper flakes. Simmer the marinara sauce for about 15 minutes, stirring occasionally.

4. Add the chopped kale to the sauce in the last 5 minutes of cooking, allowing it to wilt and integrate into the sauce.

5. Remove the spaghetti squash from the oven and let it cool slightly. Using a fork, scrape the inside of the squash to create spaghetti-like strands.

6. Serve the spaghetti squash topped with the marinara sauce and nutritional yeast and garnish with fresh basil.

Nutritional Information: Calories: 185, Protein: 6g, Carbohydrates: 30g, Fat: 8g, Fiber: 8g, Cholesterol: 0mg, Sodium: 320mg

Garlic Herb Baked Portobello Mushrooms

Ingredients

- 4 large portobello mushroom caps, cleaned and stems removed
- 4 cloves garlic, minced
- 2 tbsp extra virgin olive oil
- 1 tbsp balsamic vinegar
- 1 tsp dried thyme
- 1 tsp dried rosemary
- Salt and pepper to taste
- Fresh parsley, chopped (for garnish)

Prep Time: 10 min

Cook Time: 20 min

Serves: 4

Directions

1. Preheat the oven to 375°F (190°C). Line a baking sheet with parchment paper.

2. In a small bowl, mix together the olive oil, balsamic vinegar, minced garlic, thyme, rosemary, salt, and pepper.

3. Place the mushroom caps on the prepared baking sheet, gill side up. Brush each mushroom cap generously with the herb and garlic mixture.

4. Bake in the preheated oven for about 20 minutes, or until the mushrooms are tender and juicy.

5. Garnish with fresh parsley before serving.

Nutritional Information: Calories: 90, Protein: 2g, Carbohydrates: 6g, Fat: 7g, Fiber: 1g, Cholesterol: 0mg, Sodium: 10mg

Miso Glazed Eggplant Rounds

Ingredients

- 2 large eggplants, sliced into 1/2-inch rounds
- 3 tbsp miso paste
- 2 tbsp honey or maple syrup
- 1 tbsp rice vinegar
- 1 tbsp sesame oil
- 1 tsp ginger, grated
- 2 cloves garlic, minced
- 1 tbsp sesame seeds, for garnish
- 2 green onions, thinly sliced, for garnish

Prep Time: 10 min

Cook Time: 20 min

Serves: 4

Directions

1. Preheat your oven to 400°F (200°C) and line a baking sheet with parchment paper.

2. In a small bowl, whisk together miso paste, honey or maple syrup, rice vinegar, sesame oil, grated ginger, and minced garlic until smooth to make the glaze.

3. Arrange the eggplant rounds on the prepared baking sheet and brush each side generously with the miso glaze.

4. Bake in the preheated oven for 20 minutes, turning once halfway through, until the eggplant is tender and the glaze is caramelized.

5. Remove from oven and sprinkle with sesame seeds and green onions before serving.

Nutritional Information: Calories: 160, Protein: 3g, Carbohydrates: 21g, Fat: 7g, Fiber: 5g, Cholesterol: 0mg, Sodium: 320mg

Mushroom Risotto

 Prep Time: 10 min   Cook Time: 30 min   Serves: 4

Ingredients

- 1 cup arborio rice
- 2 cups sliced mushrooms (shiitake, maitake, and/or cremini)
- 1 small onion, finely chopped
- 2 cloves garlic, minced
- 4 cups low-sodium vegetable broth, kept warm
- 1/2 cup dry white wine (optional)
- 2 tbsp olive oil
- 1/4 cup nutritional yeast (or grated Parmesan)
- 1 tsp thyme
- Salt and black pepper to taste
- Fresh parsley, chopped

Directions

1. In a large skillet or saucepan, heat the olive oil over medium heat. Add the onion and garlic and sauté until the onion is translucent, about 5 minutes.

2. Add the mushrooms and thyme, and cook until the mushrooms are soft and browned, about 8 minutes.

3. Stir in the arborio rice, coating it with the oil and vegetable mixture. Toast the rice lightly for 2 minutes.

4. Pour in the white wine (if using), letting it absorb into the rice. Once absorbed, add a ladle of warm broth to the rice. Stir continuously until the broth is absorbed. Repeat this process, adding one ladle at a time, until the rice is creamy and al dente, about 18 minutes.

5. Remove from heat and stir in the nutritional yeast or Parmesan cheese. Season with salt and pepper to taste. Serve garnished with fresh parsley.

Nutritional Information: Calories: 340, Protein: 9g, Carbohydrates: 53g, Fat: 9g, Fiber: 4g, Cholesterol: 0mg, Sodium: 180mg

Detox Ratatouille

 Prep Time: 20 min   Cook Time: 45 min   Serves: 4

Ingredients

- 1 medium eggplant, diced
- 2 zucchinis, sliced
- 2 yellow squash, sliced
- 1 red bell pepper, chopped
- 1 yellow bell pepper, chopped
- 1 large onion, diced
- 4 cloves of garlic, minced
- 1 can (28 oz) crushed tomatoes with no added salt
- 3 tbsp extra virgin olive oil
- 1 tsp dried basil
- 1 tsp dried oregano
- 1/2 tsp thyme
- 1/2 tsp turmeric powder
- 1/4 tsp ground black pepper
- 1 small bunch of kale, stems removed and leaves chopped
- 1 tbsp apple cider vinegar
- Salt to taste
- Fresh parsley and basil for garnish

Directions

1. Preheat your oven to 375°F (190°C). In a large oven-safe dish, layer the diced eggplant, sliced zucchinis, yellow squash, chopped bell peppers, diced onion, and chopped kale. Drizzle with olive oil, apple cider vinegar, and season with salt, pepper, and turmeric.

2. In a bowl, mix the crushed tomatoes with minced garlic, dried basil, oregano, and thyme. Pour this mixture over the vegetables in the dish.

3. Cover the dish with aluminum foil and bake in the preheated oven for 40 minutes. After 40 minutes, remove the foil and continue to bake for another 5 minutes to allow some of the liquid to evaporate and the vegetables to brown slightly.

4. Remove from the oven and let it cool slightly before serving. Garnish with chopped fresh parsley and basil if desired.

Nutritional Information: Calories: 195, Protein: 6g, Carbohydrates: 33g, Fat: 8g, Fiber: 11g, Cholesterol: 0mg, Sodium: 290mg

Cauliflower Buffalo Wings

Ingredients

- 1 large head of cauliflower, cut into bite-sized florets
- 1 cup almond flour
- 1 cup water
- 1 tsp garlic powder
- 1 tsp paprika
- 1/2 tsp salt
- 1/4 tsp black pepper
- 3/4 cup hot sauce
- 1 tbsp extra virgin olive oil

Prep Time: 15 min

Cook Time: 25 min

Serves: 4

Directions

1. Preheat your oven to 450°F (230°C) and line a baking sheet with parchment paper.

2. In a large bowl, mix almond flour, water, garlic powder, paprika, salt, and black pepper to create a batter. Dip each cauliflower floret into the batter, ensuring each piece is evenly coated. Place the coated florets on the prepared baking sheet, spacing them well apart.

3. Bake in the preheated oven for 20 minutes, flipping halfway through until the batter is hardened and slightly golden.

4. While the cauliflower is baking, mix the hot sauce and olive oil in a bowl. Remove the baked florets from the oven and toss them in the hot sauce mixture to coat thoroughly.

5. Return the coated florets to the baking sheet and bake for an additional 5 minutes to set the sauce.

Nutritional Information: Calories: 180, Protein: 6g, Carbohydrates: 18g, Fat: 10g, Fiber: 5g, Cholesterol: 0mg, Sodium: 320mg

Sesame Ginger Bok Choy

Ingredients

- 4 heads of bok choy, cleaned and leaves separated
- 2 tbsp sesame oil
- 2 tsp fresh ginger, grated
- 2 cloves garlic, minced
- 2 tbsp soy sauce (or tamari for gluten-free option)
- 1 tbsp rice vinegar
- 1 tsp sesame seeds
- Red pepper flakes for heat (optional)

Prep Time: 10 min

Cook Time: 5 min

Serves: 4

Directions

1. Heat the sesame oil in a large skillet or wok over medium-high heat.

2. Add the minced garlic and grated ginger to the skillet and sauté for about 30 seconds, until fragrant.

3. Add the bok choy and toss in the oil, ginger, and garlic for about 2-3 minutes until the leaves start to wilt.

4. Stir in the soy sauce and rice vinegar, and cook for another 2 minutes until the bok choy is tender but still crisp.

5. Transfer the bok choy to a serving dish and sprinkle with sesame seeds and optional red pepper flakes.

Nutritional Information: Calories: 85, Protein: 3g, Carbohydrates: 6g, Fat: 6g, Fiber: 2g, Cholesterol: 0mg, Sodium: 510mg

Baked Sweet Potato Fries with Avocado Aioli

Ingredients

- 2 large sweet potatoes, peeled and cut into fries
- 2 tbsp olive oil
- 1 tsp smoked paprika
- 1/2 tsp garlic powder
- Salt and pepper to taste

For Avocado Aioli:
- 1 ripe avocado
- 1 clove garlic, minced
- Juice of 1 lime
- 2 tbsp olive oil
- Salt and pepper to taste

 Prep Time: 15 min

 Cook Time: 30 min

 Serves: 4

Directions

1. Preheat the oven to 425°F (220°C). Line a baking sheet with parchment paper.

2. Toss the sweet potato fries with olive oil, smoked paprika, garlic powder, salt, and pepper. Spread them in a single layer on the prepared baking sheet.

3. Bake for 30 minutes, turning halfway through, until crispy and golden brown.

4. While the fries are baking, prepare the aioli. In a blender, combine the ripe avocado, minced garlic, lime juice, olive oil, and a pinch of salt and pepper. Blend until smooth and creamy.

5. Serve the hot sweet potato fries with a side of avocado aioli for dipping.

Nutritional Information: Calories: 285, Protein: 3g, Carbohydrates: 35g, Fat: 16g, Fiber: 6g, Cholesterol: 0mg, Sodium: 120mg

Stuffed Mini Eggplant Boats with Feta Cheese

Ingredients

- 4 mini eggplants
- 1 cup cooked quinoa
- 1/2 cup cherry tomatoes, halved
- 1/2 cup cucumber, diced
- 1/4 cup feta cheese, crumbled
- 1/4 cup red onion, finely chopped
- 2 tbsp olive oil
- 1 tbsp fresh lemon juice
- 1/4 cup fresh parsley, chopped
- 1/4 cup fresh mint, chopped
- Salt and pepper to taste

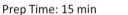 Prep Time: 15 min

 Cook Time: 30 min

 Serves: 4

Directions

1. Preheat the oven to 375°F (190°C). Cut the mini eggplants in half lengthwise and scoop out the centers to create boats, leaving about a 1/4-inch-thick shell.

2. Brush the eggplant boats with 1 tablespoon of olive oil and season with salt and pepper. Place them on a baking sheet, cut-side up, and roast in the oven for about 20-25 minutes until tender.

3. While the eggplants are roasting, in a large bowl, combine the cooked quinoa, cherry tomatoes, cucumber, red onion, feta cheese, parsley, mint, the remaining olive oil, and lemon juice. Season with salt and pepper to taste and mix well.

4. Once the eggplants are tender, remove them from the oven and fill each boat with the quinoa mixture.

5. Return the stuffed eggplants to the oven and bake for an additional 5-10 minutes, until everything is heated through.

Nutritional Information: Calories: 200, Protein: 6g, Carbohydrates: 27g, Fat: 9g, Fiber: 7g, Cholesterol: 8mg, Sodium: 180mg

Sautéed Green Beans with Almonds

Ingredients

- 1 lb fresh green beans, trimmed
- 2 tbsp extra virgin olive oil
- 1/2 cup sliced almonds
- 2 cloves garlic, minced
- 1/2 tsp turmeric powder
- 1/4 tsp ground black pepper
- 1 tbsp fresh ginger, grated
- Salt to taste
- 1 tbsp fresh lemon juice
- Fresh parsley, chopped
- 1/4 tsp cayenne pepper (optional)

 Prep Time: 10 min

 Cook Time: 12 min

 Serves: 4

Directions

1. Heat the olive oil in a large skillet over medium heat. Add the minced garlic and grated ginger, and sauté for about 1 minute until fragrant.

2. Sprinkle the turmeric and black pepper into the oil and stir to combine.

3. Add the green beans to the skillet and sauté for about 7-8 minutes, stirring occasionally, until they are tender but still have a crisp bite.

4. Stir in the sliced almonds and continue to cook for another 3-4 minutes, until the almonds are lightly toasted.

5. Season with salt and optionally, cayenne pepper, for a spicy twist. Remove from heat and squeeze the fresh lemon juice over the green beans.

6. Garnish with chopped parsley before serving.

Nutritional Information: Calories: 175, Protein: 6g, Carbohydrates: 11g, Fat: 14g, Fiber: 5g, Cholesterol: 0mg, Sodium: 7mg

Zucchini Noodles with Walnut Pesto

Ingredients

- 4 large zucchinis, spiralized
- 1 cup fresh basil leaves
- 1/2 cup walnuts, toasted
- 1/4 cup pine nuts
- 2 cloves garlic, minced
- 1/2 cup grated Parmesan cheese
- 1/2 cup extra virgin olive oil
- Juice of 1 lemon
- 1/4 tsp black pepper
- 1/3 cup grape tomatoes, halved
- Salt to taste
- 1/4 cup fresh parsley, chopped (for garnish)

 Prep Time: 20 min

 Cook Time: 0 min

 Serves: 4

Directions

1. Toast the walnuts and pine nuts in a dry skillet over medium heat until fragrant, about 3-4 minutes.

2. In a food processor, combine the toasted walnuts, pine nuts, basil leaves, minced garlic, and Parmesan cheese. Pulse until coarsely chopped.

3. While the processor is running, gradually add the olive oil, salt, black pepper and lemon juice until the pesto mixture reaches a creamy consistency.

4. Mix salt into spiralized zucchini and spread them out evenly on a kitchen towel or paper towel to soak excess water. Cover with a paper towel and squeeze as much water as possible.

5. In a large mixing bowl pour the enhanced pesto over the noodles and toss gently to coat evenly.

6. Garnish with grape tomatoes and fresh parsley.

Nutritional Information: Calories: 420, Protein: 10g, Carbohydrates: 10g, Fat: 40g, Fiber: 4g, Cholesterol: 11mg, Sodium: 190mg

Cauliflower Fried Rice

 Prep Time: 15 min   Cook Time: 10 min   Serves: 4

Ingredients

- 1 large head of cauliflower, riced
- 2 tbsp extra virgin olive oil
- 1 medium carrot, diced
- 1 red bell pepper, diced
- 1 cup broccoli florets, small
- 1 cup kale, chopped
- 1/2 cup red cabbage, shredded
- 2 green onions, sliced
- 3 cloves garlic, minced

- 1 inch piece of ginger, grated
- 1 tbsp turmeric powder
- 2 tbsp coconut aminos
- 1 tbsp apple cider vinegar
- 2 tbsp flaxseed oil
- 1/4 cup fresh cilantro, chopped
- Salt and black pepper to taste
- Hemp seeds

Directions

1. Heat the olive oil in a large skillet or wok over medium-high heat. Add the minced garlic and grated ginger, sautéing for about 1 minute until fragrant.

2. Incorporate the diced carrots, red bell peppers, broccoli florets, and red cabbage into the skillet. Cook for 3-4 minutes until they begin to soften.

3. Mix in the riced cauliflower and chopped kale. Season with salt, pepper and turmeric powder. Continue to cook for about 5 minutes, stirring occasionally, until the vegetables are tender.

4. Drizzle coconut aminos and apple cider vinegar over the cauliflower mixture, blending them evenly throughout the dish. Cook for another 2 minutes to infuse flavors.

5. Remove from heat and immediately stir in flaxseed oil to preserve the omega-3 fatty acids from heat damage.

6. Garnish with fresh cilantro and sliced green onions. Optionally, sprinkle hemp seeds on top before serving.

Nutritional Information: Calories: 205, Protein: 6g, Carbohydrates: 18g, Fat: 14g, Fiber: 6g, Cholesterol: 0mg, Sodium: 320mg

Pomegranate Balsamic Glaze Brussels Sprouts

 Prep Time: 10 min   Cook Time: 25 min   Serves: 4

Ingredients

- 1 lb Brussels sprouts, trimmed and halved
- 2 tbsp olive oil
- 3 cloves garlic, minced
- Salt and pepper to taste
- 1/2 cup pomegranate seeds

- 1/2 cup walnuts, roughly chopped
- 1 tbsp balsamic vinegar
- 1 tbsp raw honey

Directions

1. Preheat your oven to 400°F (200°C). Line a baking sheet with parchment paper.

2. Toss the Brussels sprouts with olive oil, minced garlic, salt, and pepper. Spread them out on the prepared baking sheet.

3. Roast in the preheated oven for 20-25 minutes, or until the Brussels sprouts are tender on the inside and crispy on the edges, stirring halfway through to ensure even cooking.

4. While the sprouts roast, whisk together the balsamic vinegar and honey in a small bowl. During the last 5 minutes of roasting, drizzle this glaze over the Brussels sprouts and return to the oven to finish caramelizing.

5. Remove from the oven and transfer to a serving dish. Sprinkle with pomegranate seeds and walnuts.

Nutritional Information: Calories: 210, Protein: 5g, Carbohydrates: 20g, Fat: 14g, Fiber: 6g, Cholesterol: 0mg, Sodium: 80mg

Chapter 10: Desserts

Decadent Chocolate Avocado Mousse with Pistachios

Ingredients

- 2 ripe avocados, peeled and pitted
- 1/4 cup raw cacao powder
- 1/4 cup honey or maple syrup
- 1/3 cup coconut or almond milk
- 1 tsp vanilla extract
- 1/4 cup crushed pistachios
- Pinch of sea salt

Prep Time: 15 min

Cook Time: 0 min

Serves: 4

Directions

1. Combine the avocados, cacao powder, honey (or maple syrup), coconut (or almond) milk, vanilla extract, and sea salt in a blender or food processor.

2. Blend on high until the mixture is completely smooth. Scrape down the sides as needed to ensure all ingredients are well incorporated.

3. Taste and adjust the sweetness if necessary. If the mousse is too thick, add a little more milk to reach the desired consistency.

4. Divide the mousse into serving dishes and refrigerate for at least 1 hour to set, making it thicker and more flavorful.

5. Serve chilled with crushed pistachios and a light sprinkle of sea salt.

Nutritional Information: Calories: 290, Protein: 4g, Carbohydrates: 35g, Fat: 18g, Fiber: 7g, Cholesterol: 0mg, Sodium: 30mg

Almond Butter Chocolate Chip Energy Bites

Ingredients

- 1 cup gluten-free rolled oats
- 1 cup almond butter
- 1/4 cup honey (or maple syrup)
- 1/2 cup mini chocolate chips, dairy-free if needed
- 1/4 cup ground flaxseed
- 2 tbsp chia seeds
- 1/4 tsp cinnamon powder
- 1 tsp vanilla extract
- 1/4 cup toasted coconut flakes
- Pinch of salt

Prep Time: 20 min

Cook Time: 0 min

Serves: 4

Directions

1. In a large mixing bowl, combine the rolled oats, almond butter, honey, chocolate chips, ground flaxseed, chia seeds, cinnamon, vanilla extract, and a pinch of salt. Stir until all ingredients are well combined.

2. Chill the mixture in the refrigerator for about 15 minutes to make it easier to handle.

3. Form the mixture into small balls, about the size of a walnut.

4. Roll each ball in toasted coconut flakes until well coated. Place the baking sheet in the refrigerator for 2 hours, allowing the balls to firm up.

Nutritional Information: Calories: 300, Protein: 8g, Carbohydrates: 35g, Fat: 16g, Fiber: 5g, Cholesterol: 0mg, Sodium: 40mg

Mixed Berry Crisp

Prep Time: 15 min   Cook Time: 45 min   Serves: 4

Ingredients

- 2 cups mixed berries (such as blueberries, raspberries, and strawberries), fresh or frozen
- 1 tbsp arrowroot powder (or ½ tbsp ground flax seeds)
- 2 tbsp honey or maple syrup
- 1 tsp vanilla extract
- 1 cup gluten-free oats

- 1/2 cup almond flour
- 1/4 cup chopped nuts (almonds or walnuts)
- 1/4 cup coconut oil, melted
- 1/4 cup coconut sugar
- 1/2 tsp cinnamon powder
- Pinch of salt

Directions

1. Preheat your oven to 350°F (175°C). In a mixing bowl, toss the mixed berries with arrowroot powder (or ground flax seeds), honey, and vanilla extract until well-coated. Spread the berry mixture into a greased 9-inch baking dish.

2. In another bowl, combine the gluten-free oats, almond flour, chopped nuts, melted coconut oil, coconut sugar, cinnamon, and salt. Mix until everything is well combined and crumbly.

3. Sprinkle the oat mixture evenly over the berries in the baking dish.

4. Bake in the preheated oven for 45 minutes, or until the topping is golden brown and the berries are bubbling.

5. Allow to cool slightly before serving. This dish can be enjoyed warm or at room temperature.

Nutritional Information: Calories: 350, Protein: 6g, Carbohydrates: 45g, Fat: 18g, Fiber: 6g, Cholesterol: 0mg, Sodium: 30mg

Sweet Potato Brownies

Prep Time: 15 min   Cook Time: 30 min   Serves: 4

Ingredients

- 1 medium sweet potato (about 1 cup when mashed)
- 3/4 cup almond flour
- 1/4 cup cocoa powder
- 1/2 cup maple syrup

- 1/4 cup coconut oil, melted
- 1 tsp vanilla extract
- 1/2 tsp baking powder
- 1/4 tsp salt
- 1/2 cup chopped walnuts

Directions

1. Preheat your oven to 350°F (175°C) and grease an 8x8 inch baking pan.

2. Peel and slice sweet potato into ¾ inch (or 2 cm) pieces, then steam in a steamer or steamer basket over boiling water until tender, about 20-25 minutes. Mash the cooked sweet potato in a mixing bowl.

3. Add the almond flour, cocoa powder, maple syrup, coconut oil, vanilla extract, baking powder, and salt to the mashed sweet potato. Mix until well combined.

4. Fold in the chopped walnuts if using, then spread the batter evenly into the prepared baking pan.

5. Bake in the preheated oven for 20-25 minutes or until a toothpick inserted into the center comes out clean. Allow to cool before slicing.

Nutritional Information: Calories: 367, Protein: 6g, Carbohydrates: 49g, Fat: 18g, Fiber: 7g, Cholesterol: 0mg, Sodium: 136mg

Walnut Raisin Banana Bread

Prep Time: 15 min   Cook Time: 50 min   Serves: 6

Ingredients

- 2 cups almond flour
- 3 ripe bananas, mashed
- 1/2 cup walnuts, chopped
- 1/3 cup raisins
- 1/4 cup coconut oil, melted
- 3 large eggs
- 1/4 cup honey
- 1 tsp vanilla extract
- 1 tsp baking soda
- 1/2 tsp salt
- 1/2 tsp cinnamon powder

Directions

1. Preheat your oven to 350°F (175°C) and grease a loaf pan with a bit of coconut oil.

2. In a large bowl, mix together the almond flour, baking soda, salt, and cinnamon.

3. In another bowl, whisk together the eggs, mashed bananas, honey, melted coconut oil, and vanilla extract.

4. Combine the wet ingredients with the dry ingredients and stir until well incorporated. Fold in the walnuts and raisins.

5. Pour the batter into the prepared loaf pan and smooth the top with a spatula.

6. Bake in the preheated oven for 50 minutes, or until a toothpick inserted into the center comes out clean.

7. Allow the bread to cool in the pan for 10 minutes, then transfer it to a wire rack to cool completely.

Nutritional Information: Calories: 345, Protein: 10g, Carbohydrates: 24g, Fat: 25g, Fiber: 5g, Cholesterol: 93mg, Sodium: 320mg

Banana Raspberry Nice Cream

Prep Time: 15 min   Cook Time: 0 min   Serves: 4

Ingredients

- 4 ripe bananas, peeled, sliced, and frozen
- 1 cup raspberries, fresh or frozen
- 1 cup coconut milk, full fat
- 1/4 cup fresh mint leaves
- Honey or maple syrup, to taste (optional)

Directions

1. Place the frozen banana slices, raspberries, coconut milk, and mint leaves into a blender. Blend on high until the mixture is smooth and creamy. You can add a sweetener like honey or maple syrup if desired, depending on your taste preferences and dietary needs.

2. Taste the mixture and adjust the sweetness or mintiness, if necessary. If the nice cream is too thick, add a bit more coconut milk to achieve your desired consistency.

3. Transfer the nice cream to a container and freeze for about 1-2 hours until it reaches a scoopable consistency. If you prefer a softer texture, you can serve it immediately.

4. Serve in bowls, garnish with a few fresh raspberries and mint leaves for a refreshing finish.

Nutritional Information: Calories: 230, Protein: 3g, Carbohydrates: 37g, Fat: 10g, Fiber: 5g, Cholesterol: 0mg, Sodium: 20mg

Gluten-Free Lemon Sunshine Bars

Prep Time: 20 min   Cook Time: 30 min   Serves: 6

Ingredients

For Crust:

- 1.5 cups almond flour
- 1/4 cup coconut flour
- 1/4 cup maple syrup
- 1/4 tsp sea salt
- 1/3 cup coconut oil, melted

For Filling:

- 1/3 cup maple syrup
- 4 large eggs
- Juice and zest from 2 lemons (about 1/2 cup juice)
- 1/4 cup almond milk
- 1 tbsp coconut flour
- 2 tsp vanilla extract
- 1/4 cup unsweetened shredded coconut (optional)

Directions

1. Preheat the oven to 350°F (175°C).

2. In a bowl, mix together all of crust ingredients until well combined. Press this mixture into the bottom of a greased 8x8 inch baking dish.

3. Bake the crust for 15 minutes, or until lightly golden. Remove from the oven and let cool slightly.

4. In a separate bowl, whisk together the eggs, almond milk, lemon juice, lemon zest, maple syrup, and vanilla extract. Add coconut flour last. Pour this mixture over the cooled crust.

5. Return to the oven and bake for an additional 15 minutes, or until the filling is set and no longer jiggles.

6. Remove from the oven and allow to cool completely before cutting into bars. Optionally, serve with shredded coconut.

Nutritional Information: Calories: 210, Protein: 6g, Carbohydrates: 18g, Fat: 13g, Fiber: 5g, Cholesterol: 124mg, Sodium: 120mg

Pumpkin Pie Panna Cotta with Pecans

Prep Time: 20 min   Cook Time: 10 min   Serves: 4

Ingredients

For Panna Cotta:

- 1 cup canned pumpkin puree
- 2 cups coconut milk
- 1/4 cup honey or maple syrup
- 1 tsp vanilla extract
- 1/2 tsp cinnamon powder
- 1/4 tsp nutmeg powder
- 1/4 tsp ground ginger
- 2 1/2 tsp gelatin powder
- 1/4 cup water

For Candied Pecans:

- 1/2 cup pecans, chopped
- 2 tbsp honey or maple syrup
- 1/8 tsp salt

Directions

1. In a small bowl, sprinkle gelatin over 1/4 cup of cold water and let it sit for 5 minutes to bloom.

2. In a saucepan, combine coconut milk, pumpkin puree, honey, vanilla extract, cinnamon, nutmeg, and ginger. Heat over medium heat until the mixture is warm but not boiling. Remove from heat.

3. Add the bloomed gelatin to the warm pumpkin mixture and stir until the gelatin is completely dissolved.

4. Pour the mixture into serving glasses or molds. Refrigerate for at least 4 hours, or until the panna cotta is set.

5. In a small skillet, toast the pecans over medium heat for 2-3 minutes. Add honey and salt, and continue to cook, stirring constantly, until the pecans are well coated and sticky. Spread on parchment paper to cool.

6. Sprinkle candied pecans on chilled panna cotta.

Nutritional Information: Calories: 320, Protein: 4g, Carbohydrates: 25g, Fat: 24g, Fiber: 3g, Cholesterol: 0mg, Sodium: 75mg

Baked Apples with Almond Drizzle

Prep Time: 15 min   Cook Time: 30 min   Serves: 4

Ingredients

- 4 large apples, such as Honeycrisp or Fuji, cored and sliced
- 2 tbsp coconut oil, melted
- 2 tsp cinnamon powder
- 1/4 cup almond butter, smooth

- 1 tbsp maple syrup (optional, for sweetness)
- 1 tsp vanilla extract
- Pinch of salt
- Chopped almonds, coconut flakes (optional toppings)

Directions

1. Preheat your oven to 375°F (190°C). In a large mixing bowl, toss the sliced apples with melted coconut oil and cinnamon until evenly coated.

2. Arrange the apple slices on a baking sheet lined with parchment paper. Bake in the preheated oven for about 25-30 minutes, or until the apples are soft and slightly caramelized.

3. While the apples are baking, prepare the almond butter drizzle. In a small bowl, combine almond butter, maple syrup (if using), vanilla extract, and a pinch of salt. Stir until smooth and well combined.

4. Once the apples are done, remove them from the oven and let them cool slightly. Drizzle the almond butter mixture over the warm apples.

5. Serve immediately, garnished with optional chopped almonds and coconut flakes if desired.

Nutritional Information: Calories: 210, Protein: 2g, Carbohydrates: 28g, Fat: 11g, Fiber: 5g, Cholesterol: 0mg, Sodium: 55mg

Chocolate Coconut Truffles

Prep Time: 15 min   Cook Time: 0 min   Serves: 4

Ingredients

- 1 cup gluten-free dark chocolate chips (at least 70% cacao)
- 1/2 cup coconut cream
- 1 tsp coconut oil
- 1/4 tsp cardamom powder

- 1/8 tsp cayenne pepper
- 1/2 cup unsweetened shredded coconut (for coating)
- A pinch of sea salt

Directions

1. In a small saucepan, combine dark chocolate chips, coconut cream, and coconut oil. Heat over a low flame, stirring constantly until the mixture is smooth.

2. Remove from heat and stir in the cardamom, cayenne pepper, and a pinch of sea salt.

3. Transfer the mixture to a bowl and let it cool to room temperature. Once cooled, cover and refrigerate for about 1 hour or until the mixture is firm enough to handle.

4. Scoop out teaspoon-sized portions of the chilled mixture and roll into balls. Roll each ball in shredded coconut to coat thoroughly.

5. Place the coated truffles on a parchment-lined tray and refrigerate until firm, about 30 minutes, before serving.

Nutritional Information: Calories: 210, Protein: 2g, Carbohydrates: 18g, Fat: 15g, Fiber: 3g, Cholesterol: 0mg, Sodium: 20mg

Mangolicious Matcha Chia Parfait

Prep Time: 15 min   Cook Time: 0 min   Serves: 4

Ingredients

- 1/4 cup chia seeds
- 1 cup unsweetened almond milk
- 1 tbsp matcha powder
- 1 tbsp honey (or maple syrup)
- 1 tsp vanilla extract
- 1 large ripe mango, peeled and diced
- 1/2 cup macadamia nuts, toasted and roughly chopped
- Fresh mint leaves for garnish (optional)

Directions

1. In a mixing bowl, combine the chia seeds, almond milk, matcha powder, honey, and vanilla extract. Whisk until the matcha is fully dissolved. Let the mixture sit for about 10 minutes, then stir again to prevent clumping. Cover and refrigerate for at least 4 hours or overnight until it achieves a pudding-like consistency.

2. Once the chia pudding is set, prepare the parfait. Spoon a layer of matcha chia pudding into four glasses. Add a layer of diced mango over the pudding.

3. Sprinkle a layer of toasted macadamia nuts over the mango. Repeat the layering if desired or based on the size of your glasses.

4. Garnish with fresh mint leaves before serving for an added touch of freshness.

Nutritional Information: Calories: 245, Protein: 4g, Carbohydrates: 29g, Fat: 15g, Fiber: 7g, Cholesterol: 0mg, Sodium: 45mg

Lemon Blueberry Cheesecake Bars

Prep Time: 20 min   Cook Time: 35 min   Serves: 6

Ingredients

- 1 1/2 cups almond flour
- 1/4 cup coconut oil, melted
- 2 tbsp honey
- 1/4 tsp sea salt
- 2 cups raw cashews, soaked for 4 hours and drained
- 1/2 cup canned coconut milk
- 1/2 cup lemon juice, freshly squeezed
- 1/3 cup maple syrup
- Zest of 1 lemon
- 1 tsp vanilla extract
- 1 cup fresh blueberries
- Lemon slices and additional blueberries for garnish (optional)

Directions

1. Preheat the oven to 350°F (175°C). Line an 8x8-inch baking dish with parchment paper.

2. Make the crust: In a bowl, mix almond flour, coconut oil, honey, vanilla extract, and sea salt. Press the mixture into the bottom of the prepared dish. Bake for 10 minutes, then remove and let cool slightly.

3. In a high-powered blender, blend soaked cashews, coconut milk, lemon juice, maple syrup, and lemon zest until smooth and creamy.

4. Pour the cashew mixture over the cooled crust and smooth the top with a spatula. Scatter the fresh blueberries evenly across the top.

5. Bake in the preheated oven for 25 minutes, or until the filling is set.

6. Allow the bars to cool at room temperature, then refrigerate for at least 3 hours before slicing into bars.

7. Garnish with lemon slices and additional blueberries if desired.

Nutritional Information: Calories: 325, Protein: 7g, Carbohydrates: 35g, Fat: 20g, Fiber: 4g, Cholesterol: 0mg, Sodium: 15mg

Golden Spice Energy Balls

 Prep Time: 20 min   Cook Time: 0 min   Serves: 6

Ingredients

- 1 cup dates, pitted
- 1 cup gluten-free oats
- 1/4 cup almond butter
- 2 tbsp turmeric powder
- 1/2 cup unsweetened coconut flakes
- 1 tbsp chia seeds
- 1 tsp cinnamon powder
- 1/2 tsp ginger powder
- A pinch of black pepper
- 1 tbsp lemon zest

Directions

1. Place the pitted dates in a food processor and blend until they form a sticky base.

2. Add gluten-free oats, almond butter, turmeric powder, cinnamon, ginger, and black pepper to the food processor. Blend until the mixture is thoroughly combined and sticky.

3. Transfer the mixture to a bowl, add chia seeds and lemon zest, and mix well.

4. Scoop out tablespoon-sized portions of the mixture and roll into balls.

5. Roll each ball in coconut flakes until evenly coated.

6. Refrigerate for at least 45 minutes to firm up, allowing the flavors to meld beautifully.

Nutritional Information: Calories: 160, Protein: 5g, Carbohydrates: 25g, Fat: 8g, Fiber: 5g, Cholesterol: 0mg, Sodium: 12mg

Quinoa Chocolate Chip Cookies

 Prep Time: 15 min   Cook Time: 12 min   Serves: 4

Ingredients

- 1 cup cooked quinoa, cooled
- 1/2 cup almond butter
- 1/2 cup pure maple syrup
- 1/2 cup dark chocolate chips, dairy-free if needed
- 1/4 cup coconut oil, melted
- 1 tsp vanilla extract
- 1/2 tsp baking soda
- 1/2 tsp sea salt
- 1 egg or 1 flax egg (1 tbsp ground flaxseed mixed with 3 tbsp water, let sit for 5 minutes)

Directions

1. Preheat the oven to 350°F (175°C) and line a baking sheet with parchment paper.

2. In a large bowl, mix together the cooked quinoa, almond butter, and baking soda.

3. Add the flax egg (or regular egg), melted coconut oil, maple syrup, and vanilla extract to the dry ingredients and mix until well combined.

4. Fold in chocolate chips and a pinch of sea salt.

5. Scoop tablespoon-sized portions of dough onto the prepared baking sheet, flattening slightly, and bake for 10-12 minutes or until golden brown around the edges. Let cool on the baking sheet for a few minutes before transferring to a wire rack to cool completely.

Nutritional Information: Calories: 160, Protein: 3g, Carbohydrates: 18g, Fat: 9g, Fiber: 2g, Cholesterol: 0mg, Sodium: 100mg

Avocado Lime Tart

 Prep Time: 20 min   Cook Time: 0 min   Serves: 6

Ingredients

For Crust:

- 1 1/2 cups almonds
- 1 cup Medjool dates, pitted
- 1/4 tsp sea salt
- 1 tbsp coconut oil, melted

For Filling:

- 2 ripe avocados
- 1/2 cup fresh lime juice
- 1/2 cup honey or maple syrup
- 1/2 cup coconut cream
- 1 tsp lime zest
- 1 tsp vanilla extract

Directions

1. In a food processor, blend almonds until they are finely ground. Add dates, sea salt, and melted coconut oil, and process until the mixture is sticky and holds together when pressed.

2. Press the almond-date mixture firmly into the bottom and sides of a tart pan to form the crust. Place the crust in the freezer to set while you prepare the filling.

3. In a blender or food processor, combine the avocados, lime juice, honey (or maple syrup), coconut cream, lime zest, and vanilla extract. Blend until the mixture is smooth and creamy.

4. Pour the avocado-lime filling into the chilled almond-date crust. Smooth the top with a spatula. Chill the tart in the refrigerator for at least 2 hours, or until set.

Nutritional Information: Calories: 320, Protein: 5g, Carbohydrates: 35g, Fat: 20g, Fiber: 7g, Cholesterol: 0mg, Sodium: 80mg

Choco-Tropical Macaroons

 Prep Time: 20 min   Cook Time: 20 min   Serves: 4

Ingredients

- 2 cups unsweetened shredded coconut
- 1/2 cup pure maple syrup
- 2 tsp vanilla extract
- 2 egg whites
- 1/4 tsp salt
- 1/4 cup finely chopped dried pineapple
- 1/4 cup dark chocolate chips
- 1 tbsp chia seeds
- 1 tbsp lemon zest
- 1/3 tsp ginger powder

Directions

1. Preheat your oven to 325°F (165°C) and line a baking sheet with parchment paper and grease it with a little coconut oil.

2. In a large bowl, combine the shredded coconut, maple syrup, vanilla extract, chopped dried pineapple, dark chocolate chips, chia seeds, lemon zest, and ginger.

3. In a separate bowl, beat the egg whites and salt until soft peaks form. Gently fold the beaten egg whites into the coconut mixture until fully combined.

4. Using a spoon or small ice cream scoop, drop spoonfuls of the mixture onto the prepared baking sheet, spacing them about 2 inches apart. Slightly shape them into mounds.

5. Bake for 18-20 minutes or until the macaroons are golden brown. Allow them to cool on the baking sheet for a few minutes before transferring to a wire rack to cool completely.

Nutritional Information: Calories: 270, Protein: 3g, Carbohydrates: 32g, Fat: 15g, Fiber: 4g, Cholesterol: 0mg, Sodium: 100mg

Berry Bliss Coconut Popsicles

 Prep Time: 20 min

 Cook Time: 4 hours (freezing)

 Serves: 4

Ingredients

- 1/2 cup fresh blueberries
- 1/2 cup fresh raspberries
- 1 cup creamy coconut milk
- 2 tbsp chia seeds
- 2 tbsp agave nectar (maple syrup or honey)
- 1 tsp pure vanilla extract
- 1 cup coconut yogurt
- 1/2 cup toasted crushed almonds
- 1 tbsp shredded coconut (optional, for extra crunch)

Directions

1. In a blender, combine raspberries, blueberries, creamy coconut milk, chia seeds, agave nectar, and vanilla extract. Blend until smooth.

2. Pour the mixture into popsicle molds, leaving a little space at the top. Insert sticks and freeze for at least 4 hours or until they are solid.

3. Once frozen, remove popsicles from molds. Dip each popsicle into coconut yogurt, ensuring an even and generous coating.

4. Roll the yogurt-coated popsicles in toasted crushed almonds and shredded coconut, making sure every bite is packed with flavor. Place them on a baking sheet lined with parchment paper and freeze for an additional 30 minutes.

Nutritional Information: Calories: 190, Protein: 4g, Carbohydrates: 16g, Fat: 13g, Fiber: 5g, Cholesterol: 0mg, Sodium: 10mg

Salted Caramel Peanut Butter Nice Cream

 Prep Time: 15 min

 Cook Time: 10 min

 Serves: 4

Ingredients

- 4 ripe bananas, sliced and frozen
- 2 tbsp natural peanut butter
- 1/4 cup unsweetened almond milk
- 6 Medjool dates, pitted
- 1/4 tsp sea salt
- 1/4 cup water
- 2 tbsp cocoa nibs
- 1/2 tsp cinnamon powder
- 1/4 tsp cayenne pepper
- 1/2 cup pecans
- 2 tbsp maple syrup
- 1/2 tsp smoked paprika

Directions

1. Blend frozen bananas, peanut butter, and almond milk in a food processor until smooth and creamy.

2. For the caramel, blend dates, sea salt, and water until smooth. Stir in cinnamon and cayenne pepper.

3. To make the spicy candied pecans, toss pecans with maple syrup and smoked paprika. Spread on a baking sheet and bake at 350°F (175°C) for 10 minutes or until caramelized.

4. Serve nice cream in bowls, drizzle with date caramel, sprinkle with cocoa nibs, and top with spicy candied pecans.

Nutritional Information: Calories: 320, Protein: 6g, Carbohydrates: 58g, Fat: 12g, Fiber: 8g, Cholesterol: 0mg, Sodium: 160mg

Double Chocolate Zucchini Bread

Prep Time: 20 min | Cook Time: 50 min | Serves: 6

Ingredients

- 1 1/2 cups gluten-free oat flour
- 1/2 cup raw cacao powder
- 1 tsp baking soda
- 1/2 tsp sea salt
- 1/4 tsp cinnamon powder
- 1/2 cup unsweetened applesauce
- 1/2 cup coconut oil, melted
- 1 cup finely grated zucchini
- 2 large eggs
- 1 tsp pure vanilla extract
- 1/2 cup dark chocolate chips

For Espresso Glaze:
- 1 cup powdered monk fruit sweetener
- 1-2 tbsp freshly brewed espresso
- 1-2 tbsp coconut milk

Directions

1. Preheat your oven to 350°F (175°C). Line a 9x5 inch loaf pan with parchment paper and grease it with a little coconut oil.

2. In a bowl, mix together the oat flour, raw cacao powder, baking soda, sea salt, and cinnamon.

3. In another larger bowl, whisk together the applesauce, melted coconut oil, grated zucchini, eggs, and vanilla extract until well combined. Slowly add the dry ingredients to the wet ingredients. Fold in the dark chocolate chips.

4. Pour the batter into the prepared loaf pan, smoothing the top with a spatula. Bake in the preheated oven for about 50 minutes, or until a toothpick inserted in the center comes out clean.

5. For the glaze, whisk together monk fruit sweetener, espresso, and coconut milk until smooth. Adjust the consistency with more coconut milk if needed.

6. Allow the bread to cool in the pan for 10 minutes, then remove and cool completely on a wire rack. Drizzle the espresso glaze over the top before serving.

Nutritional Information: Calories: 295, Protein: 8g, Carbohydrates: 38g, Fat: 15g, Fiber: 6g, Cholesterol: 62mg, Sodium: 300mg

Zesty Pistachio Ginger Cookies

Prep Time: 20 min | Cook Time: 12 min | Serves: 6

Ingredients

- 1 cup almond flour
- 1/4 cup coconut flour
- 1/4 cup honey or maple syrup
- 1/4 cup coconut oil, melted
- 1 tbsp grated fresh ginger
- Zest of 1 lemon
- 1/2 tsp baking soda
- 1/4 tsp salt
- 1/4 cup finely chopped crystallized ginger
- 2 tbsp chia seeds
- 1/4 cup finely chopped pistachios
- 1 tsp vanilla extract

Directions

1. Preheat your oven to 350°F (175°C) and line a baking sheet with parchment paper.

2. In a medium bowl, whisk together almond flour, coconut flour, baking soda, salt, chia seeds, and chopped pistachios.

3. In a separate bowl, mix honey or maple syrup, melted coconut oil, grated ginger, lemon zest, crystallized ginger, and vanilla extract until well combined.

4. Combine wet and dry ingredients, stirring until a vibrant dough forms. Scoop tablespoon-sized portions onto the prepared baking sheet, flattening slightly.

5. Bake for 12 minutes or until edges are golden and centers are set. Cool on the baking sheet for 5 minutes before transferring to a wire rack.

Nutritional Information: Calories: 160, Protein: 4g, Carbohydrates: 18g, Fat: 11g, Fiber: 3g, Cholesterol: 0mg, Sodium: 60mg

Chapter 11: Smoothies

Green Detox Smoothie

Ingredients

- 1 cup spinach, fresh
- 1 cup kale, fresh
- 1 medium cucumber, peeled and chopped
- 1 green apple, cored and chopped
- Juice of 1 lemon
- 1-inch piece of ginger, peeled and minced
- 1 ½ cups coconut water
- Ice cubes (optional)

Prep Time: 10 min

Cook Time: 0 min

Serves: 2

Directions

1. Wash the spinach and kale thoroughly to remove any dirt or grit.
2. Peel and chop the cucumber and green apple into small pieces suitable for blending.
3. Peel and mince the ginger.
4. Place all the ingredients into a blender, adding the lemon juice and coconut water last.
5. Blend on high until all ingredients are thoroughly combined and the mixture is smooth. Add ice cubes if desired. Adjust the amount of coconut water to achieve your desired smoothie consistency.

Nutritional Information: Calories: 150, Protein: 4g, Carbohydrates: 35g, Fat: 1g, Fiber: 6g, Cholesterol: 0mg, Sodium: 250mg

Ginger Beet Smoothie

Ingredients

- 1 medium beet, peeled and chopped
- 2 medium carrots, peeled and chopped
- 1-inch piece of fresh ginger, peeled
- 1 small apple
- 1 tbsp chia seeds
- 1/8 tsp cayenne pepper
- 2 cups water or coconut water
- 1 tbsp lemon juice
- Stevia for additional sweetness (optional)
- Ice cubes (optional)

Prep Time: 10 min

Cook Time: 0 min

Serves: 2

Directions

1. Place the chopped beet, carrots, apple and ginger into a blender.
2. Add the chia seeds, cayenne pepper, water or coconut water, and lemon juice to the blender.
3. Blend on high speed until the mixture is smooth and well combined.
4. Add stevia if using and blend again to incorporate. Taste and adjust sweetness if necessary.
5. If desired, add ice cubes and blend until smooth. Serve immediately.

Nutritional Information: Calories: 95, Protein: 2g, Carbohydrates: 21g, Fat: 1g, Fiber: 5g, Cholesterol: 0mg, Sodium: 106mg

Minty Matcha De-stress Smoothie

Ingredients

- 2 scoops plant-based protein powder (sugar-free)
- 1 cup fresh spinach, washed
- 10-12 fresh mint leaves
- 1 ripe banana, peeled
- 2 cups unsweetened almond milk
- 1 tsp matcha green tea powder
- Ice cubes (optional)

 Prep Time: 10 min

 Cook Time: 0 min

 Serves: 4

Directions

1. Place the plant-based protein powder, fresh spinach, mint leaves, and banana in a blender.

2. Add the unsweetened almond milk and matcha green tea powder to the blender.

3. Blend all ingredients on high speed until smooth and creamy, ensuring no chunks remain.

4. Taste the smoothie and adjust the sweetness or intensity of the matcha by adding more banana or matcha powder if desired.

5. Pour into glasses and serve immediately for the freshest flavor.

Nutritional Information: Calories: 240, Protein: 18g, Carbohydrates: 24g, Fat: 7g, Fiber: 4g, Cholesterol: 0mg, Sodium: 180mg

Berry Blast Immunity Smoothie

Ingredients

- 1 cup frozen mixed berries (strawberries, blueberries, raspberries, blackberries)
- 2 cups fresh spinach, washed
- 1 small avocado
- 1-2 inches fresh ginger, chopped
- 2 tbsp ground flaxseed
- 2 cups coconut water
- 2 tbsp apple cider vinegar
- 1 tbsp chia seeds
- Juice of 1 lemon
- 2-3 tsp honey (or maple syrup)

 Prep Time: 12 min

 Cook Time: 0 min

 Serves: 2

Directions

1. Combine frozen berries, avocado, spinach, ginger, ground flaxseed, and chia seeds in a blender.

2. Add coconut water, honey (or maple syrup), apple cider vinegar, and lemon juice to the mixture.

3. Blend on high until the smoothie is completely smooth and the ingredients are thoroughly mixed. Add more coconut or filtered water if thinner consistency is desired.

4. Taste and add a bit more lemon juice if a sharper flavor is desired. Add more honey (or maple syrup) if more sweetness is desired.

5. Serve immediately in chilled glasses for a revitalizing and health-boosting drink.

Nutritional Information: Calories: 180, Protein: 4g, Carbohydrates: 34g, Fat: 3g, Fiber: 8g, Cholesterol: 0mg, Sodium: 100mg

Cleansing Watermelon Basil Smoothie

Ingredients

- 4 cups watermelon, cubed and seedless
- 1 cup spinach, fresh
- 10 basil leaves, fresh
- 1 tbsp lime juice, freshly squeezed
- 1 cup coconut water
- 1 tbsp chia seeds
- 1-2 inches fresh ginger, shopped
- 1/2 cucumber, sliced

Prep Time: 15 min

Cook Time: 0 min

Serves: 4

Directions

1. Add the watermelon, spinach, basil leaves, chopped ginger, sliced cucumber, and chia seeds to a blender.

2. Pour in freshly squeezed lime juice and coconut water.

3. Blend on high speed until everything is smooth and fully combined.

4. Taste and adjust the ingredients as desired. If you prefer a thinner smoothie, you can add more coconut water.

5. Serve the smoothie fresh or chilled, garnished with a few basil leaves or a lime wheel for an extra zing.

Nutritional Information: Calories: 82, Protein: 2g, Carbohydrates: 18g, Fat: 1g, Fiber: 3g, Cholesterol: 0mg, Sodium: 40mg

Tropical Gold Smoothie

Ingredients

- 3 Medjool dates, pitted
- 1/2 tsp turmeric powder
- 1 ripe banana
- 1/2 cup pineapple chunks
- 1/2 cup mango chunks
- 1 cup coconut milk
- 1 cup filtered water (or 1 additional cup of coconut milk)
- A pinch of black pepper

Prep Time: 10 min

Cook Time: 0 min

Serves: 2

Directions

1. Place the pitted dates in a small bowl and cover with warm water. Let them soak for about 5 minutes to soften.

2. In a blender, combine the softened dates, turmeric powder, banana, pineapple, mango, coconut milk and filtered water.

3. Blend on high until the mixture is smooth and creamy.

4. Add a pinch of black pepper and blend for a few more seconds to mix thoroughly.

5. Pour into glasses and serve immediately for the best flavor and nutrient retention.

Nutritional Information: Calories: 240, Protein: 3g, Carbohydrates: 35g, Fat: 11g, Fiber: 4g, Cholesterol: 0mg, Sodium: 20mg

Crimson Glow Smoothie

Ingredients

- 1 cup fresh or frozen cherries, pitted
- 1 cup pomegranate juice
- 1 medium beet, peeled and chopped
- 1 ripe banana
- 1 scoop plant-based protein powder (vanilla or unflavored)
- 1 tbsp honey or maple syrup (optional)
- 1 cup ice cubes

Prep Time: 10 min

Cook Time: 0 min

Serves: 4

Directions

1. Place the cherries, pomegranate juice, chopped beet, and banana into a blender.
2. Add plant-based protein powder and honey, if using, and blend on high until smooth.
3. Toss in the ice cubes and blend again until the mixture is frosty and smooth.
4. Taste the smoothie and adjust sweetness if desired.
5. Pour into glasses and serve immediately.

Nutritional Information: Calories: 160, Protein: 10g, Carbohydrates: 33g, Fat: 2g, Fiber: 5g, Cholesterol: 0mg, Sodium: 40mg

Blueberry Nut Recovery Smoothie

Ingredients

- 1 cup unsweetened almond milk
- 1/2 cup fresh or frozen blueberries
- 2 tbsp almond butter
- 2 tbsp ground flaxseed
- 1 scoop plant-based protein powder (preferably vanilla or unflavored)
- Ice cubes (optional)

Prep Time: 5 min

Cook Time: 0 min

Serves: 2

Directions

1. Place the almond milk, blueberries, almond butter, ground flaxseed, and plant-based protein powder into a blender.
2. Add a few ice cubes if a thicker consistency is desired.
3. Blend on high until smooth and creamy.
4. Pour into glasses and serve immediately for optimal freshness and flavor.

Nutritional Information: Calories: 280, Protein: 18g, Carbohydrates: 20g, Fat: 16g, Fiber: 5g, Cholesterol: 0mg, Sodium: 180mg

Ginger Muscle Soother Smoothie

Ingredients

- 2 tbsp almond butter
- 3 inches fresh ginger root, peeled and grated
- 1 medium banana, sliced
- 1/2 tsp turmeric powder
- A pinch of black pepper
- 2 scoops plant-based protein powder (preferably vanilla or unflavored)
- 2 cups unsweetened almond milk
- 1 tsp chia seeds
- 1 tbsp flaxseed oil
- A handful of spinach

Prep Time: 12 min

Cook Time: 0 min

Serves: 2

Directions

1. Place the grated ginger, banana, turmeric powder, black pepper, and spinach in a blender. Add a small amount of almond milk to facilitate blending.

2. Add the almond butter, plant-based protein powder, chia seeds, and flaxseed oil to the blender.

3. Pour in the rest of the almond milk and blend on high until the mixture is completely smooth, which might take about 2-3 minutes depending on your blender.

4. Taste the smoothie and adjust the ginger or turmeric according to your preference for more spiciness or a stronger anti-inflammatory effect.

5. Serve the smoothie immediately, or keep it chilled for up to an hour to preserve the freshness and nutritional quality.

Nutritional Information: Calories: 395, Protein: 22g, Carbohydrates: 35g, Fat: 21g, Fiber: 8g, Cholesterol: 0mg, Sodium: 185mg

Choco-Banana Recharge Smoothie

Ingredients

- 2 ripe bananas, peeled
- 2 tbsp almond butter
- 4 dates, pitted
- 2 tbsp unsweetened cacao powder
- 1 scoop plant-based protein powder
- 1 cup unsweetened almond milk
- 1 cup filtered water
- 1 tbsp chia seeds

Prep Time: 10 min

Cook Time: 0 min

Serves: 2

Directions

1. Place the bananas, almond butter, and dates in a blender. Blend until the mixture is smooth.

2. Add the unsweetened cacao powder and plant-based protein powder to the blender. Blend again until all ingredients are well incorporated.

3. Pour in the almond milk and add the chia seeds. Blend on high speed until the smoothie reaches a creamy consistency.

4. Divide the smoothie between two glasses and serve immediately for optimal freshness and nutrient retention.

Nutritional Information: Calories: 380, Protein: 15g, Carbohydrates: 53g, Fat: 14g, Fiber: 10g, Cholesterol: 0mg, Sodium: 170mg

Protein Power Smoothie

Ingredients

- 1 cup cooked green lentils
- 2 cups fresh spinach leaves
- 1 ripe avocado, peeled and pitted
- 1 green apple, cored and chopped
- 2 scoops of protein powder (plant-based preferred)
- 2 cups almond milk (or any preferred plant-based milk)
- 4 dates, pitted
- 1 tbsp chia seeds
- 1 tbsp honey (optional, for sweetness)
- 1 cup ice cubes

Prep Time: 10 min   Cook Time: 0 min   Serves: 4

Directions

1. Add the cooked lentils, spinach leaves, avocado, green apple, protein powder, almond milk, and dates to a blender.

2. Blend until smooth and creamy.

3. Add the chia seeds, honey, and ice cubes to the blender.

4. Taste the smoothie and adjust the thickness if desired. If it's too thick, add a bit more almond milk.

5. Blend again until the ice is crushed and the smoothie is well mixed. Pour into glasses and enjoy immediately.

Nutritional Information: Calories: 350, Protein: 22g, Carbohydrates: 48g, Fat: 14g, Fiber: 14g, Cholesterol: 0mg, Sodium: 150mg

Papaya Energy Smoothie

Ingredients

- 1 cup papaya, peeled and diced
- 1-inch piece of fresh ginger, peeled and grated
- 2 cups fresh spinach leaves
- 2 cups coconut water
- Juice of 1 lime
- 1 tbsp chia seeds
- 1 scoop vanilla protein powder (preferably plant-based)

Prep Time: 10 min   Cook Time: 0 min   Serves: 4

Directions

1. Combine the papaya, ginger, spinach, coconut water, lime juice, chia seeds, and protein powder in a blender.

2. Blend on high until smooth and creamy.

3. Taste and adjust lime juice or coconut water if necessary.

4. Pour into glasses and serve immediately.

Nutritional Information: Calories: 180, Protein: 15g, Carbohydrates: 28g, Fat: 4g, Fiber: 5g, Cholesterol: 5mg, Sodium: 80mg

Avocado Kale Vitality Smoothie

Ingredients

- 1 ripe avocado, peeled and pitted
- 2 cups kale leaves, stems removed
- 1 cucumber, peeled and chopped
- 1/2 cup fresh mint leaves
- 2 cups coconut water
- 1 tbsp chia seeds
- 1 tbsp fresh lemon juice
- 1 tsp grated ginger
- Ice cubes (optional)

Prep Time: 10 min

Cook Time: 0 min

Serves: 4

Directions

1. Combine avocado, kale, cucumber, mint, and coconut water in a blender.
2. Add chia seeds, lemon juice, and ginger to the blender.
3. Blend on high speed until smooth and creamy, adding ice cubes if desired for a colder smoothie.
4. Pour into glasses and serve immediately.

Nutritional Information: Calories: 190, Protein: 3g, Carbohydrates: 20g, Fat: 12g, Fiber: 8g, Cholesterol: 0mg, Sodium: 100mg

Raspberry Mint Sparkler Smoothie

Ingredients

- 1 cup fresh raspberries
- 1 cup sparkling water
- 1 cup unsweetened almond milk
- 1 cup spinach leaves
- 1/2 cup Greek yogurt
- 1 tbsp chia seeds
- 1 tbsp fresh mint leaves
- 1 tbsp honey (optional)
- 1 tsp freshly grated ginger
- Ice cubes

Prep Time: 10 min

Cook Time: 0 min

Serves: 4

Directions

1. In a blender, combine raspberries, almond milk, spinach, Greek yogurt, chia seeds, mint leaves, honey (if using), and grated ginger.
2. Blend until smooth, adding ice cubes to achieve desired consistency.
3. Pour the smoothie into glasses, leaving some space at the top.
4. Slowly add sparkling water to each glass, stirring gently to combine.

Nutritional Information: Calories: 110, Protein: 6g, Carbohydrates: 16g, Fat: 3g, Fiber: 4g, Cholesterol: 4mg, Sodium: 50mg

Sweet Potato Mango Fusion Smoothie

Ingredients

- 1 medium sweet potato, cooked and cooled
- 1/2 cup mango chunks (fresh or frozen)
- 1 cup unsweetened almond milk
- 1/2 cup Greek yogurt
- 1 tbsp honey or maple syrup
- 1/2 tsp cinnamon powder
- 1/4 tsp ginger powder
- 1/4 tsp nutmeg powder
- 1/2 tsp vanilla extract
- 1 cup ice cubes

Prep Time: 10 min   Cook Time: 15 min   Serves: 4

Directions

1. Peel the cooked sweet potato and cut it into chunks.

2. In a blender, combine the sweet potato chunks, mango chunks, almond milk, Greek yogurt, honey or maple syrup, cinnamon, ginger, nutmeg, and vanilla extract.

3. Blend until smooth and creamy.

4. Add ice cubes and blend again until the smoothie is thick and chilled.

5. Pour into glasses and serve immediately.

Nutritional Information: Calories: 155, Protein: 5g, Carbohydrates: 29g, Fat: 2g, Fiber: 4g, Cholesterol: 5mg, Sodium: 60mg

Liver Detox Smoothie

Ingredients

- 2 cups dandelion greens, washed and chopped
- 1 banana, sliced
- 1 cup pineapple chunks
- 1 cup coconut water
- 1 tbsp chia seeds
- 1 tbsp honey (optional)
- 1 tsp fresh ginger, grated
- 1 cup ice cubes

Prep Time: 10 min   Cook Time: 0 min   Serves: 4

Directions

1. Place the dandelion greens, banana, pineapple chunks, coconut water, chia seeds, honey, and ginger in a blender.

2. Blend on high speed until smooth and creamy.

3. Add ice cubes and blend again until the ice is fully incorporated and the smoothie is cold.

4. Pour into glasses and serve immediately.

Nutritional Information: Calories: 130, Protein: 2g, Carbohydrates: 30g, Fat: 2g, Fiber: 5g, Cholesterol: 0mg, Sodium: 50mg

Firestarter Pineapple Smoothie

Ingredients

- 2 cups fresh pineapple chunks
- 1 cup coconut water
- 1 jalapeño, seeds removed and chopped
- 1/4 cup fresh mint leaves
- 1 banana
- 1 scoop protein powder (preferably plant-based)
- 1 tbsp hemp seeds
- 1 tbsp flax seeds
- 1 tbsp honey (optional)
- Ice cubes (optional)

Prep Time: 10 min

Cook Time: 0 min

Serves: 4

Directions

1. Combine pineapple chunks, coconut water, chopped jalapeño, fresh mint leaves, banana, protein powder, hemp seeds, flax seeds, and honey in a blender.
2. Blend on high until smooth and creamy. Add ice cubes if a colder smoothie is desired, and blend again until smooth.
3. Taste and adjust sweetness if needed by adding more honey.
4. Pour into glasses and serve immediately.

Nutritional Information: Calories: 150, Protein: 10g, Carbohydrates: 22g, Fat: 4g, Fiber: 4g, Cholesterol: 0mg, Sodium: 50mg

Chai Spice Butternut Squash Smoothie

Ingredients

- 1 cup butternut squash puree
- 1 banana
- 1 cup unsweetened almond milk
- 1/2 cup Greek yogurt
- 1 tbsp honey or maple syrup
- 1/2 tsp cinnamon powder
- 1/4 tsp nutmeg powder
- 1/4 tsp ginger powder
- 1/4 tsp cardamom powder
- 1 tsp vanilla extract
- 1 tbsp maca powder
- 1 tbsp chia seeds
- 1 tbsp almond butter
- 3 pitted dates
- 1 cup ice cubes

Prep Time: 10 min

Cook Time: 0 min

Serves: 4

Directions

1. Add the butternut squash puree, banana, almond milk, Greek yogurt, honey, cinnamon, nutmeg, ginger, cardamom, vanilla extract, maca powder, chia seeds, almond butter, dates, and ice cubes to a blender.
2. Blend on high speed until smooth and creamy.
3. Taste and adjust sweetness if needed by adding more honey or maple syrup.
4. Pour into glasses and serve immediately.

Nutritional Information: Calories: 210, Protein: 6g, Carbohydrates: 38g, Fat: 6g, Fiber: 5g, Cholesterol: 5mg, Sodium: 75mg

Bloody Mary Smoothie

Prep Time: 12 min

Cook Time: 0 min

Serves: 4

Ingredients

- 2 cups tomato juice
- 1 cup diced cucumber
- 1 cup diced celery
- 1/2 cup diced red bell pepper
- 1/4 cup lemon juice
- 1/4 cup apple cider vinegar
- 1/4 tsp cayenne pepper powder
- 1/4 tsp sea salt
- 1/4 tsp black pepper
- 1/2 tsp smoked paprika
- 1/2 tsp turmeric powder
- 1/4 cup fresh parsley, chopped
- 1/2 cup kale or spinach leaves, chopped
- 1/2 cup ice cubes
- Celery stalks for garnish (optional)

Directions

1. Add tomato juice, cucumber, celery, red bell pepper, lemon juice, apple cider vinegar, fresh parsley, and kale or spinach leaves to a blender.

2. Add soy sauce, cayenne pepper, sea salt, black pepper, smoked paprika, and turmeric to the blender.

3. Blend until smooth, then add ice cubes and blend again until the mixture is cold and well combined.

4. Pour into glasses and garnish with fresh parsley or celery stalks if desired.

Nutritional Information: Calories: 70, Protein: 3g, Carbohydrates: 14g, Fat: 0.5g, Fiber: 4g, Cholesterol: 0mg, Sodium: 350mg

High-Protein PB&J Smoothie

Prep Time: 5 min

Cook Time: 0 min

Serves: 4

Ingredients

- 2 cups frozen strawberries
- 2 bananas
- 1/2 cup natural peanut butter
- 2 cups almond milk (or milk of choice)
- 1 scoop vanilla protein powder
- 1 tbsp honey (optional)
- 1 tsp vanilla extract

Directions

1. Place frozen strawberries, bananas, peanut butter, almond milk, protein powder, honey, and vanilla extract in a blender.

2. Blend on high speed until smooth and creamy.

3. Taste and adjust sweetness with additional honey if desired.

4. Pour into glasses and serve immediately.

Nutritional Information: Calories: 380, Protein: 25g, Carbohydrates: 45g, Fat: 18g, Fiber: 6g, Cholesterol: 0mg, Sodium: 200mg

Chapter 12: Sides & Snacks

Roasted Garlic Hummus with Veggie Sticks

Ingredients

- 1 large head of garlic
- 1 can (15 oz) chickpeas, drained and rinsed
- 3 tbsp tahini
- 2 tbsp fresh lemon juice
- 1/4 cup olive oil, plus extra for roasting garlic
- 1/2 tsp cumin powder
- Salt to taste
- Freshly ground black pepper to taste
- Assorted veggie sticks (carrots, celery, cucumber, bell peppers), for serving

 Prep Time: 15 min

 Cook Time: 40 min

 Serves: 4

Directions

1. Preheat the oven to 400°F (200°C). Slice the top off the head of garlic to expose the cloves. Drizzle with a little olive oil, wrap in aluminum foil, and roast in the oven for about 40 minutes, or until the cloves are soft and golden.

2. Squeeze the roasted garlic cloves out of their skins into a food processor. Add the chickpeas, tahini, lemon juice, 1/4 cup olive oil, and cumin. Season with salt and pepper.

3. Process until the mixture is perfectly smooth, adding a few tablespoons of water if needed to reach the desired consistency.

4. Taste and adjust the seasoning, adding more salt, pepper, or lemon juice if needed.

5. Serve the hummus in a bowl, accompanied by an array of fresh veggie sticks.

Nutritional Information: Calories: 295, Protein: 8g, Carbohydrates: 24g, Fat: 20g, Fiber: 6g, Cholesterol: 0mg, Sodium: 290mg

Crispy Baked Parmesan Zucchini Chips

Ingredients

- 4 medium zucchinis, thinly sliced
- 1/2 cup grated Parmesan cheese
- 1/4 cup almond flour
- 1 tsp garlic powder
- 1/2 tsp black pepper
- 1/4 tsp salt
- Olive oil spray

 Prep Time: 15 min

 Cook Time: 25 min

 Serves: 4

Directions

1. Preheat your oven to 425°F (220°C) and line a baking sheet with parchment paper.

2. In a small bowl, mix together Parmesan cheese, almond flour, garlic powder, salt, and pepper.

3. Arrange zucchini slices in a single layer on the baking sheet. Lightly spray the zucchini with olive oil spray.

4. Sprinkle the Parmesan mixture evenly over the zucchini slices.

5. Bake in the preheated oven for 25 minutes, or until the zucchini is golden and crispy.

Nutritional Information: Calories: 120, Protein: 8g, Carbohydrates: 10g, Fat: 7g, Fiber: 3g, Cholesterol: 10mg, Sodium: 240mg

Savory Sweet Potato Toast

Ingredients

- 2 large sweet potatoes, cut into 1/2-inch-thick slices
- 1/4 cup almond butter or any nut butter of your choice
- 1 ripe avocado, mashed (optional)
- 1/4 cup hummus (optional)
- Sliced radishes, pumpkin seeds, a sprinkle of chia seeds, or a drizzle of olive oil (optional toppings)
- Salt and pepper

Prep Time: 10 min

Cook Time: 25 min

Serves: 4

Directions

1. Preheat your oven to 400°F (200°C). Line a baking sheet with parchment paper.

2. Arrange sweet potato slices in a single layer on the baking sheet. Bake for 15 minutes, flip each slice, and continue baking for another 10 minutes or until slices are tender and slightly crispy on the edges.

3. Remove the sweet potato slices from the oven and let them cool slightly.

4. To assemble, spread a layer of nut butter on the sweet potato slices; other good substitutes are hummus and mashed avocado. Add any optional toppings as desired.

5. Season with salt and pepper to taste before serving.

Nutritional Information: Calories: 210, Protein: 6g, Carbohydrates: 34g, Fat: 8g, Fiber: 6g, Cholesterol: 0mg, Sodium: 180mg

Cucumber Avocado Rolls

Ingredients

- 2 large cucumbers
- 1 ripe avocado, mashed
- 1/2 red bell pepper, finely diced
- 1/2 cup sprouts (alfalfa or broccoli)
- 2 tbsp nutritional yeast
- 1/2 tsp smoked paprika
- Salt and pepper

Prep Time: 15 min

Cook Time: 0 min

Serves: 4

Directions

1. Using a mandoline or a sharp knife, slice the cucumbers lengthwise into thin strips.

2. In a small bowl, mix the mashed avocado with nutritional yeast, smoked paprika, salt, and pepper until well combined.

3. Lay the cucumber strips flat on a clean surface, and spread a thin layer of the avocado mixture over each strip.

4. Sprinkle diced bell peppers and sprouts evenly across each cucumber strip.

5. Carefully roll each cucumber strip tightly to encase the filling. Secure with a toothpick if necessary.

Nutritional Information: Calories: 110, Protein: 4g, Carbohydrates: 13g, Fat: 7g, Fiber: 5g, Cholesterol: 0mg, Sodium: 45mg

Coconut-Crusted Tofu Bites

Prep Time: 15 min

Cook Time: 25 min

Serves: 4

Ingredients

- 14 oz block of firm tofu, pressed and cut into cubes
- 1/2 cup unsweetened shredded coconut
- 1/4 cup almond flour
- 1 tsp garlic powder
- 1 tsp paprika
- 1/2 tsp salt
- 1/4 tsp black pepper
- 1 tbsp coconut oil, melted
- 2 tbsp soy sauce or tamari (for a gluten-free option)
- 1 tbsp lime juice

Directions

1. Preheat your oven to 400°F (200°C) and line a baking sheet with parchment paper.

2. In a shallow bowl, mix the shredded coconut, almond flour, garlic powder, paprika, salt, and black pepper.

3. In another bowl, combine the melted coconut oil, soy sauce, and lime juice.

4. Dip each tofu cube first in the liquid mixture, then roll in the coconut mixture to coat evenly. Place the coated tofu cubes on the prepared baking sheet.

5. Bake in the preheated oven for 25 minutes, turning halfway through, until the coating is golden and crispy.

Nutritional Information: Calories: 210, Protein: 12g, Carbohydrates: 9g, Fat: 15g, Fiber: 4g, Cholesterol: 0mg, Sodium: 430mg

Spicy Chickpea Snack Mix

Prep Time: 10 min

Cook Time: 30 min

Serves: 4

Ingredients

- 1 cup chickpeas, drained and rinsed
- 1/2 cup raw almonds
- 1/2 cup raw pumpkin seeds
- 1/2 cup raw sunflower seeds
- 1 tbsp olive oil
- 1 tsp smoked paprika
- 1/2 tsp garlic powder
- 1/2 tsp cayenne pepper
- 1/2 tsp turmeric powder
- 1/2 tsp sea salt

Directions

1. Preheat your oven to 375°F (190°C). Pat the chickpeas dry with a paper towel to remove any excess moisture.

2. In a large bowl, combine the chickpeas, almonds, pumpkin and sunflower seeds. Drizzle with olive oil and toss until evenly coated.

3. Sprinkle smoked paprika, garlic powder, cayenne pepper, turmeric, and sea salt over the chickpea mix. Toss again to distribute the spices evenly.

4. Spread the mixture in a single layer on a baking sheet lined with parchment paper.

5. Roast in the preheated oven for about 30 minutes, stirring halfway through, until the chickpeas are golden and crispy.

Nutritional Information: Calories: 250, Protein: 9g, Carbohydrates: 21g, Fat: 15g, Fiber: 6g, Cholesterol: 0mg, Sodium: 300mg

Roasted Garlic Mashed Cauliflower

Ingredients

- 1 large head of cauliflower, cut into florets
- 4 cloves of garlic, peeled
- 2 tbsp olive oil
- 1/4 cup unsweetened almond milk
- 1 tbsp nutritional yeast (optional for a cheesy flavor)
- 1 tsp fresh lemon juice
- Salt and pepper to taste
- 1 tbsp fresh chives, chopped (optional)
- 1/4 tsp smoked paprika (optional for a smoky flavor)

Prep Time: 10 min

Cook Time: 20 min

Serves: 4

Directions

1. Preheat oven to 400°F (200°C). Toss cauliflower florets and garlic cloves with olive oil, salt, and pepper. Spread on a baking sheet.

2. Roast in the preheated oven for 20 minutes, or until cauliflower is tender and golden brown.

3. Transfer roasted cauliflower and garlic to a food processor. Add almond milk, nutritional yeast, lemon juice, and blend until smooth and creamy. Adjust seasoning with salt, pepper, and smoked paprika as needed.

4. Serve hot, garnished with fresh chives for a burst of color and flavor.

Nutritional Information: Calories: 90, Protein: 4g, Carbohydrates: 10g, Fat: 4.5g, Fiber: 4g, Cholesterol: 0mg, Sodium: 60mg

Spiced Carrot Fries with Avocado Dip

Ingredients

- 6 large carrots, peeled and cut into fries
- 2 tbsp olive oil
- 1 tsp turmeric powder
- 1/2 tsp garlic powder
- Salt and black pepper to taste
- 1 ripe avocado
- 1/4 cup plain Greek yogurt
- 1 tbsp lime juice
- 1 clove garlic, minced
- 1 tbsp fresh cilantro, chopped

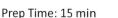

Prep Time: 15 min

Cook Time: 25 min

Serves: 4

Directions

1. Preheat your oven to 425°F (220°C). Line a baking sheet with parchment paper.

2. In a large bowl, toss the carrot fries with olive oil, turmeric, garlic powder, salt, and black pepper until well coated. Spread the carrots in a single layer on the prepared baking sheet.

3. Roast in the preheated oven for 25 minutes, turning once halfway through, until crispy and golden.

4. While the carrots are roasting, prepare the dipping sauce. In a blender, combine the avocado, Greek yogurt, lime juice, minced garlic, and cilantro. Blend until smooth and creamy.

5. Serve the roasted carrot fries hot with the creamy avocado dipping sauce on the side.

Nutritional Information: Calories: 200, Protein: 4g, Carbohydrates: 27g, Fat: 10g, Fiber: 6g, Cholesterol: 1mg, Sodium: 120mg

Seed-Crusted Sweet Potato Wedges

Ingredients

- 2 large sweet potatoes, peeled and cut into wedges
- 1/4 cup ground flaxseeds
- 1/4 cup sesame seeds
- 2 tbsp sunflower seeds, crushed
- 2 large eggs, beaten
- 1 tsp ground cumin
- 1 tsp ground turmeric
- Salt and black pepper
- 1/2 cup fresh cilantro, finely chopped
- Zest and juice of 2 limes
- 1 tbsp honey
- 1/4 cup Greek yogurt (use non-dairy options if desired)

Prep Time: 20 min

Cook Time: 25 min

Serves: 4

Directions

1. Preheat the oven to 400°F (200°C). Line a baking sheet with parchment paper.

2. In a shallow dish, combine flaxseeds, sesame seeds, sunflower seeds, cumin, turmeric, salt, and pepper. In another dish, place the beaten eggs.

3. Dip each sweet potato wedge first in the egg, then in the seed mixture, pressing to coat well. Place the wedges on the prepared baking sheet.

4. Bake for 25 minutes, or until golden and crispy, turning halfway through.

5. While the wedges are baking, in a small bowl, mix together the cilantro, lime zest and juice, honey, and yogurt.

6. Serve the crispy sweet potato wedges hot with the yogurt sauce on the side.

Nutritional Information: Calories: 295, Protein: 6g, Carbohydrates: 33g, Fat: 17g, Fiber: 6g, Cholesterol: 93mg, Sodium: 200mg

Maple Syrup Roasted Brussels Sprouts

Ingredients

- 1.5 pounds Brussels sprouts, trimmed and halved
- 2 tbsp olive oil
- 2 tbsp maple syrup
- 2 tbsp Dijon mustard
- 1/2 tsp salt
- 1/4 tsp black pepper
- 1/4 tsp garlic powder

Prep Time: 10 min

Cook Time: 25 min

Serves: 4

Directions

1. Preheat your oven to 400°F (200°C) and line a baking sheet with parchment paper.

2. In a large bowl, whisk together olive oil, maple syrup, Dijon mustard, salt, black pepper, and garlic powder.

3. Add the Brussels sprouts to the bowl and toss to coat evenly with the mustard maple mixture.

4. Spread the Brussels sprouts in a single layer on the prepared baking sheet.

5. Roast in the preheated oven for 25 minutes, stirring halfway through, until they are caramelized and tender.

Nutritional Information: Calories: 158, Protein: 3g, Carbohydrates: 20g, Fat: 8g, Fiber: 4g, Cholesterol: 0mg, Sodium: 330mg

Turmeric Ginger Broccoli Bites

Prep Time: 15 min   Cook Time: 25 min   Serves: 4

Ingredients

- 4 cups of broccoli florets
- 2 tbsp extra virgin olive oil
- 1 1/2 tsp turmeric powder
- 1 1/2 tsp ground ginger
- 1/2 tsp ground black pepper
- 1/4 tsp Himalayan pink salt
- A sprinkle of sesame seeds (for garnish)
- Fresh cilantro or parsley, finely chopped (for garnish)

For Tahini Dipping Sauce:
- 1/4 cup tahini
- 1/4 ripe avocado
- 1 tbsp lemon juice
- 1 clove garlic, minced
- 2 tbsp warm water
- 1 tsp honey or maple syrup (optional)
- Salt and freshly ground black pepper

Directions

1. Preheat your oven to 400 degrees F (200 degrees C).

2. In a large bowl, combine the broccoli florets with olive oil, turmeric, ginger, black pepper, and pink salt. Toss well to ensure the florets are evenly coated.

3. Arrange the broccoli on a baking sheet in a single layer. Roast in the preheated oven for about 20 minutes, or until the edges are crispy and the florets are tender.

4. For the dipping sauce, blend tahini, avocado, lemon juice, minced garlic, warm water, and honey (if using) in a blender until smooth. Season with salt and pepper to taste.

5. Serve the roasted broccoli warm, sprinkled with sesame seeds and fresh herbs. Accompany with the creamy tahini-avocado sauce for dipping.

Nutritional Information: Calories: 215, Protein: 7g, Carbohydrates: 17g, Fat: 16g, Fiber: 6g, Cholesterol: 0mg, Sodium: 85mg

Spicy Cauliflower Popcorn

Prep Time: 15 min   Cook Time: 25 min   Serves: 4

Ingredients

- 1 medium head cauliflower, cut into bite-sized florets
- 2 tbsp extra virgin olive oil
- 2 tbsp sriracha sauce
- 1 tsp turmeric powder
- 1 tsp smoked paprika
- 1 tsp cumin powder
- ½ tsp garlic powder
- ½ tsp onion powder
- ½ tsp ground ginger
- ½ tsp black pepper
- Salt to taste
- 1 tbsp fresh lemon juice
- Zest of one lemon
- 1 tbsp chopped fresh parsley (optional)

Directions

1. Preheat your oven to 400°F (200°C). Line a baking sheet with parchment paper.

2. In a large bowl, mix olive oil, avocado oil, sriracha sauce, turmeric, smoked paprika, cumin, garlic powder, onion powder, ground ginger, black pepper, salt, lemon juice, and lemon zest until well combined.

3. Toss cauliflower florets in the spicy, detoxifying marinade, coating them thoroughly. Spread them on the prepared baking sheet in a single layer.

4. Roast in the preheated oven for 20-25 minutes, flipping halfway through, until the cauliflower is golden, crisp on the edges, and tender.

5. For extra flavor and freshness, sprinkle with chopped fresh parsley before serving.

Nutritional Information: Calories: 140, Protein: 3g, Carbohydrates: 14g, Fat: 8g, Fiber: 5g, Cholesterol: 0mg, Sodium: 240mg

Anti-Inflammatory Kale Chips

Ingredients

- 1 bunch kale, washed and dried
- 2 tbsp olive oil
- 1/4 cup nutritional yeast
- 1/2 tsp Himalayan pink salt
- 1/2 tsp turmeric powder
- 1/4 tsp garlic powder
- 1/4 tsp onion powder
- 1/8 tsp black pepper

 Prep Time: 10 min

 Cook Time: 20 min

 Serves: 4

Directions

1. Preheat your oven to 300°F (150°C). Line a baking sheet with parchment paper.

2. Remove the kale leaves from the stems and tear them into bite-sized pieces. Place the kale pieces in a large bowl.

3. Drizzle olive oil over the kale and add salt, turmeric, garlic powder, onion powder, and black pepper. Toss well to evenly coat the kale.

4. Sprinkle nutritional yeast over the coated kale, tossing again to distribute it evenly.

5. Spread the kale in a single layer on the prepared baking sheet. Bake in the preheated oven for 20 minutes, or until the edges are crisp but not burnt, turning halfway through.

Nutritional Information: Calories: 150, Protein: 6g, Carbohydrates: 10g, Fat: 10g, Fiber: 4g, Cholesterol: 0mg, Sodium: 300mg

Edamame Guacamole

Ingredients

- 1 cup shelled edamame (boiled or steamed)
- 2 ripe avocados, peeled and pitted
- 1/4 cup cilantro leaves
- 1 small jalapeño, seeded and diced
- 1 clove garlic, minced
- 1/4 cup red onion, finely chopped
- Juice of 1 lime
- Salt and black pepper

 Prep Time: 10 min

 Cook Time: 5 min

 Serves: 4

Directions

1. Blend edamame, avocados, cilantro, jalapeño, garlic, and lime juice in a food processor or blender until smooth.

2. Transfer the mixture to a bowl and fold in the chopped red onion.

3. Season with salt and black pepper to taste.

4. Serve with fresh vegetable sticks or gluten-free tortilla chips for a healthy, anti-inflammatory snack.

Nutritional Information: Calories: 180, Protein: 6g, Carbohydrates: 14g, Fat: 12g, Fiber: 7g, Cholesterol: 0mg, Sodium: 90mg

Healing Spice Acorn Rings

Ingredients

- 1 large acorn squash, washed and sliced into ½-inch rings (seeds removed)
- 2 tbsp extra virgin olive oil
- 2 tbsp pure maple syrup
- 1/2 tsp turmeric powder
- 1/2 tsp cinnamon powder
- 1/4 tsp ginger powder
- 1/4 tsp cayenne pepper (optional, for a hint of heat)
- 1 tsp finely grated lemon zest
- Pinch of sea salt
- Fresh parsley, chopped (for garnish)

Prep Time: 10 min

Cook Time: 25 min

Serves: 4

Directions

1. Preheat your oven to 400°F (200°C) and line a baking sheet with parchment paper.
2. Arrange the acorn squash rings on the baking sheet.
3. In a large bowl, mix olive oil, maple syrup, sea salt, cinnamon, turmeric, ginger, cayenne pepper (if using), and lemon zest.
4. Coat squash rings with the mix ensuring each piece is coated evenly.
5. Bake for 20-25 minutes or until the squash rings are tender and caramelized at the edges. Flip them halfway through for even cooking.
6. Garnish with chopped fresh parsley before serving for an added burst of flavor.

Nutritional Information: Calories: 165, Protein: 2g, Carbohydrates: 25g, Fat: 6g, Fiber: 4g, Cholesterol: 0mg, Sodium: 60mg

Gluten-free Tabbouleh

Ingredients

- 1 medium head cauliflower, grated (or 4 cups of cauliflower rice)
- 1 cup diced tomatoes
- 1 cup diced cucumber
- 1/2 cup chopped parsley
- 1/4 cup chopped mint leaves
- 1/4 cup lemon juice
- 3 tbsp olive oil
- Salt and black pepper

Prep Time: 15 min

Cook Time: 5 min

Serves: 4

Directions

1. In a large skillet over medium heat, lightly sauté the grated cauliflower in 1 tablespoon of olive oil for 3-5 minutes, just until tender. Set aside to cool.
2. In a large mixing bowl, combine the diced tomatoes, cucumber, parsley, and mint leaves.
3. Add the cooled cauliflower to the bowl and drizzle with lemon juice and remaining olive oil. Season with salt and black pepper to taste, then toss well to combine.
4. Refrigerate the tabbouleh for at least 30 minutes before serving to allow the flavors to meld together.

Nutritional Information: Calories: 150, Protein: 3g, Carbohydrates: 12g, Fat: 10g, Fiber: 4g, Cholesterol: 0mg, Sodium: 120mg

Garlic Sautéed Kale

Prep Time: 5 min   Cook Time: 10 min   Serves: 4

Ingredients

- 1 large bunch of kale, stems removed and leaves torn into pieces
- 2 tbsp extra virgin olive oil
- 2 tbsp avocado oil
- 4 cloves garlic, minced
- 1 lemon, zested and juiced
- 1 avocado, diced
- 1 tsp smoked paprika
- 1 tsp cumin powder
- 1/2 tsp crushed red pepper flakes (or to taste)
- Salt and black pepper

Directions

1. In a large skillet, heat the olive oil and avocado oil over medium heat.

2. Add the minced garlic to the skillet and sauté for about 1 minute until fragrant.

3. Add the smoked paprika, cumin, and crushed red pepper flakes to the garlic, stirring for about 30 seconds to bloom the spices.

4. Add the torn kale leaves to the skillet and stir to coat them with oil and spices. Cook for 5-7 minutes, stirring frequently, until the kale is wilted and tender.

5. Drizzle with lemon juice, sprinkle with lemon zest, and season with salt and black pepper. Toss to combine.

6. Remove from heat and gently fold in the diced avocado for a creamy finish. Serve warm.

Nutritional Information: Calories: 180, Protein: 4g, Carbohydrates: 12g, Fat: 14g, Fiber: 5g, Cholesterol: 0mg, Sodium: 180mg

Baked BBQ Plantain Chips

Prep Time: 10 min   Cook Time: 15 min   Serves: 4

Ingredients

- 2 large green plantains
- 1 tbsp olive oil
- 1 tsp smoked paprika
- 1 tsp garlic powder
- 1 tsp onion powder
- 1 tsp chili powder
- 1/2 tsp salt
- 1/2 tsp black pepper

Directions

1. Preheat your oven to 400°F (200°C). Line a baking sheet with parchment paper or a silicone baking mat.

2. Peel the plantains and slice them into thin rounds, about 1/8 inch thick. Place the slices in a large mixing bowl.

3. Drizzle olive oil over the plantain slices and toss to coat. In a small bowl, mix together smoked paprika, garlic powder, onion powder, chili powder, salt, and pepper. Sprinkle the spice mixture over the plantains and toss until evenly coated.

4. Arrange the seasoned plantain slices in a single layer on the prepared baking sheet. Bake for 12-15 minutes or until they are crispy and golden brown, flipping once halfway through to ensure even cooking.

5. Remove the chips from the oven and let them cool slightly before serving..

Nutritional Information: Calories: 140, Protein: 1g, Carbohydrates: 30g, Fat: 3g, Fiber: 2g, Cholesterol: 0mg, Sodium: 120mg

Eggplant Fries with Marinara Sauce

Prep Time: 15 min   Cook Time: 25 min   Serves: 4

Ingredients

- 2 medium eggplants
- 1 cup almond flour
- 1/2 cup grated Parmesan cheese
- 2 large eggs
- 1 tsp garlic powder

- 1 tsp paprika
- 1 tsp dried oregano
- Salt and pepper
- 1 cup marinara sauce (store-bought or homemade see pg. 71)

Directions

1. Preheat the oven to 425°F (220°C). Line a baking sheet with parchment paper and lightly spray with cooking spray.

2. Slice the eggplants into fry-shaped sticks. In a bowl, mix almond flour, Parmesan cheese, garlic powder, paprika, dried oregano, salt, and pepper. In another bowl, beat the eggs.

3. Dip each eggplant stick into the beaten eggs, then coat with the almond flour mixture. Place on the prepared baking sheet in a single layer.

4. Lightly spray the coated eggplant sticks with cooking spray. Bake for 20-25 minutes, turning halfway, until golden and crispy. Serve with warmed marinara sauce.

Nutritional Information: Calories: 250, Protein: 10g, Carbohydrates: 25g, Fat: 12g, Fiber: 7g, Cholesterol: 60mg, Sodium: 400mg

Herb-Crusted Avocado Wedges

Prep Time: 15 min   Cook Time: 15 min   Serves: 4

Ingredients

- 2 ripe avocados, halved, pitted, and sliced into wedges
- 1/2 cup almond flour
- 1 tsp dried oregano
- 1 tsp dried thyme
- 1 tsp turmeric powder
- 1 tsp smoked paprika
- 1 tsp garlic powder

- 1/4 tsp cayenne pepper
- 1/2 tsp sea salt
- 1/4 tsp black pepper
- 2 large eggs, beaten
- 1 tbsp avocado oil (for greasing the baking sheet)
- Fresh cilantro and lime wedges for garnish

Directions

1. Preheat your oven to 425°F (220°C) and lightly grease a baking sheet with avocado oil.

2. Slice the avocados in half, remove the pit, and carefully cut each half into 4-6 wedges.

3. In a shallow bowl, mix almond flour, turmeric powder, smoked paprika, garlic powder, oregano, thyme, cayenne pepper (if using), black pepper and sea salt.

4. Dip each avocado wedge in the beaten eggs, ensuring a good coating. Then, roll the wedges in the almond flour mixture, pressing gently to ensure the coating adheres. Place each wedge on the prepared baking sheet.

5. Bake for 12-15 minutes, turning halfway through, until the wedges are crispy and golden. For extra crispiness, broil the fries for 1-2 minutes at the end.

6. Garnish with fresh cilantro leaves and lime wedges.

Nutritional Information: Calories: 280, Protein: 6g, Carbohydrates: 14g, Fat: 22g, Fiber: 10g, Cholesterol: 0mg, Sodium: 180mg

Chapter 13:
Embracing the Lifestyle

When people think of reducing inflammation, they often focus on food choices. While an anti-inflammatory diet is foundational, lifestyle changes beyond nutrition can further improve overall well-being. Incorporating other lifestyle adjustments such as quality sleep, regular exercise, and stress reduction can bolster your body's resilience against chronic inflammation. Moreover, keeping a health journal is a valuable tool for tracking progress and maintaining motivation.

Incorporating Anti-Inflammatory Lifestyle Changes

An anti-inflammatory lifestyle integrates healthy habits that reduce chronic inflammation and protect against disease. These changes address the underlying causes of inflammation, bringing about a more holistic transformation. By adopting mindful movement practices and creating environments that promote calm, small, incremental adjustments can lead to significant improvements. Regularly writing down your daily habits, emotions, and how you feel physically in a health journal can reveal patterns and provide clarity about the lifestyle choices that work best for you.

The Importance of Sleep, Exercise, and Stress Reduction

- **Sleep:** Quality sleep is essential for immune system function and cellular repair. Lack of sleep disrupts hormone levels like cortisol and melatonin, which contribute to inflammation. Aim for 7-9 hours of quality sleep per night. Develop a consistent bedtime routine, keep your room dark and cool, avoid eating heavy meals and limit screen time before bed to improve sleep quality. Record your nightly sleep hours and morning energy levels in your health journal to identify trends.

- **Exercise:** Physical activity reduces inflammation by promoting blood flow, maintaining a healthy weight, and releasing anti-inflammatory cytokines. Moderate, consistent exercise like walking, swimming, or yoga has been shown to reduce inflammation markers. Aim for 30 minutes a day, 5 days a week. Choose enjoyable activities to stay motivated long-term. Log your workouts and post-exercise energy levels to celebrate progress and make adjustments.

- **Stress Reduction:** Chronic stress triggers inflammation through elevated stress hormones. Techniques like meditation, deep breathing, or progressive muscle relaxation can counteract these effects. Hobbies, connecting with loved ones, or spending time in nature also reduce stress. Reflecting on daily stressors in your journal can help identify triggers and track how different relaxation techniques impact your mood.

Chapter 14:
Overcoming Common Challenges

Starting an anti-inflammatory diet is a powerful step towards transforming your health, but it can come with its own set of challenges. The path to reducing inflammation through dietary choices is filled with incredible potential for improved well-being, yet navigating the changes can be daunting. From figuring out what foods to eat to overcoming cravings and adjusting meal plans, it's normal to encounter obstacles along the way. However, with the right strategies, you can make this transition smoother and more enjoyable. Below are some of the tips and practical advice to help you conquer these challenges and fully embrace the benefits of an anti-inflammatory lifestyle.

- **Rewiring Your Palate:** Processed foods train the brain to crave hyper-palatable flavors. Break free by incorporating bitter greens like arugula or dandelion into your diet to reset your taste buds. Additionally, fermented foods like sauerkraut or kefir not only deliver probiotics but also recalibrate your cravings through gut-brain signaling.

- **Addressing Nutrient Deficiencies:** A poorly balanced diet can lead to lingering fatigue, muscle cramps, or brain fog. Balance your intake by focusing on magnesium (found in pumpkin seeds and dark chocolate), vitamin D (fatty fish), and zinc (nuts and seeds). Nutritional deficiencies can undermine progress, so regular blood tests to identify gaps are advisable.

- **Leveraging Food Synergies:** Some foods work best when paired strategically. Curcumin in turmeric needs piperine from black pepper to enhance absorption. Similarly, fat-soluble vitamins in leafy greens require healthy fats like avocado or olive oil to unlock their benefits. Pair your ingredients mindfully to maximize their anti-inflammatory properties.

- **Breaking Routine Monotony:** If your meals feel repetitive, branch out with new anti-inflammatory recipes like buckwheat porridge or mung bean salad. Integrate herbs and spices that aren't in your regular rotation, such as fenugreek or sumac, to keep your meals fresh and flavorful.

- **Managing Emotional Eating:** Stress can trigger emotional eating, undermining your diet. Develop non-food coping mechanisms like journaling, yoga, or taking a brisk walk. Evening rituals like lighting candles or playing calming music can also shift your mindset away from food as a crutch.

- **Finding Hidden Inflammatory Culprits:** Watch out for sneaky ingredients like added sugars in salad dressings or inflammatory oils in processed snacks. Opt for homemade versions or diligently read labels, prioritizing products with whole-food ingredients and minimal additives.

Practice Holistic Approach to Reduce Inflammation

- **Mindful Eating:** Eating should be a pleasant, unhurried experience. Practice mindful eating by savoring each bite, chewing thoroughly, and avoiding distractions like screens while dining. This helps improve digestion and nutrient absorption. Use your journal to track food choices and how you feel after meals.

- **Toxin Reduction:** Environmental toxins exacerbate inflammation. Opt for natural cleaning products, avoid processed foods with additives, and use high-quality, fragrance-free personal care products. Write down the changes you make and how they impact your symptoms.

- **Social Connections:** Positive social connections can mitigate inflammation by boosting oxytocin, reducing stress hormones, and providing a support network. Engage in meaningful conversations and activities with friends, family, or community groups. Track your social engagements to see how they correlate with your mood and energy.

- **Hydration:** Drinking enough water helps flush out toxins and lubricate joints. Start your day with a glass of water and carry a bottle to stay hydrated. Use a health journal to note daily water intake and its impact on your energy levels.

- **Grounding Practices:** Spending time outdoors barefoot or lying on the grass can help balance the body's electromagnetic field, reducing inflammation and promoting relaxation. Record how grounding practices influence your stress levels over time.

By integrating these lifestyle changes with a nourishing diet, you will unlock the full potential of a holistic approach to reducing inflammation. Treat your adjustments as a journey rather than a race. With patience, consistency, and an open mind, you will find that these changes naturally blend into your daily routine, providing a sustainable path toward optimal health. Your health journal will become a powerful tool for self-discovery and tracking your progress.

Chapter 15:
The 28-Day Clean Meal Plan

Week-by-Week Guide

WEEK 1

BREAKFAST	Spinach and Mushroom Breakfast Hash (p.21)	Choco-Banana Recharge Smoothie (p.113)	Goat Cheese Spinach Omelet (p.30)	Chia and Pumpkin Seed Pudding (p.21)	Spinach and Mushroom Breakfast Hash (p.21)	Choco-Banana Recharge Smoothie (p.113)	Chia and Pumpkin Seed Pudding (p.21)
LUNCH	Lentil and Roasted Beet Salad (p.33)	Pesto Rubbed Halibut with Roasted Tomatoes (leftover)	Hearty Gluten-free Minestrone (leftover)	Spinach and Feta Stuffed Chicken Breasts (leftover)	Stuffed Bell Peppers with Lentils and Walnuts (leftover)	Smoky Chickpeas and Kale Roasted Salmon (leftover)	Turmeric Chicken Skewers (leftover)
DINNER	Pesto Rubbed Halibut with Roasted Tomatoes (p.62)	Hearty Gluten-free Minestrone (p.47)	Spinach and Feta Stuffed Chicken Breasts (p.66)	Stuffed Bell Peppers with Lentils and Walnuts (p.89)	Smoky Chickpeas and Kale Roasted Salmon (p.55)	Turmeric Chicken Skewers (p.64)	Rainbow Vegetarian Chili (p.45)
SNACK	Roasted Garlic Hummus with Veggie Sticks (p.119)	Savory Sweet Potato Toast (p.120)	Roasted Garlic Hummus with Veggie Sticks (p.119)	Almond Butter Chocolate Chip Energy Bites (p.99)	Savory Sweet Potato Toast (p.120)	Roasted Garlic Hummus with Veggie Sticks (p.119)	Almond Butter Chocolate Chip Energy Bites (p.99)

WEEK 2

BREAKFAST	Almond Flour Pancakes with Blueberries (p.22)	Zucchini and Carrot Fritters (p.24)	Breakfast Apple Bake (p.26)	Zesty Papaya Smoothie (p.114)	Almond Flour Pancakes with Blueberries (p.22)	Zucchini and Carrot Fritters (p.24)	Breakfast Apple Bake (p.26)
LUNCH	Rainbow Vegetarian Chili (leftover)	Baked Cod with Crispy Garlic Broccoli (leftover)	Spiced Lamb with Veggies and Raisins (leftover)	Healing Tomato and Sardine Stew (leftover)	Stuffed Mini Eggplant Boats with Feta Cheese (leftover)	Supercharged Chicken and Veggie Stir-Fry (leftover)	Macadamia Cod with Mango-Mint Salsa (leftover)
DINNER	Baked Cod with Crispy Garlic Broccoli (p.53)	Spiced Lamb with Veggies and Raisins (p.79)	Healing Tomato and Sardine Stew (p.48)	Stuffed Mini Eggplant Boats with Feta Cheese (p.95)	Supercharged Chicken and Veggie Stir-Fry (p.73)	Macadamia Cod with Mango-Mint Salsa (p.62)	Spaghetti Squash with Marinara Sauce (p.91)
SNACK	Crispy Baked Tahini Cauliflower Bites (p.91)	Decadent Chocolate Avocado Mousse with Pistachios (p.99)	Spiced Carrot Fries with Avocado Dip (p.122)	Decadent Chocolate Avocado Mousse with Pistachios (p.99)	Crispy Baked Parmesan Zucchini Chips (p.119)	Spiced Carrot Fries with Avocado Dip (p.122)	Crispy Baked Tahini Cauliflower Bites (p.91)

WEEK 3

BREAKFAST	Berry Blast Immunity Smoothie (p.110)	Zucchini and Red Pepper Frittata (p.23)	Pumpkin Spice Muffins (p.29)	Zucchini and Red Pepper Frittata (p.23)	Berry Blast Immunity Smoothie (p.110)	Zucchini and Red Pepper Frittata (p.23)	Pumpkin Spice Muffins (p.29)
LUNCH	Spaghetti Squash with Marinara Sauce (leftover)	Grilled Salmon and Asparagus Salad (leftover)	Spicy Peanut Butter Chicken Lettuce Wraps (leftover)	Clams Stir-Fry with Bell Peppers (leftover)	Healing Spice Chicken with Apricots (leftover)	Lamb Chops with Rosemary Mint Pesto (leftover)	Detox Ratatouille (leftover)
DINNER	Grilled Salmon and Asparagus Salad (p.35)	Spicy Peanut Butter Chicken Lettuce Wraps (p.75)	Clams Stir-Fry with Bell Peppers (p.60)	Healing Spice Chicken with Apricots (p.66)	Lamb Chops with Rosemary Mint Pesto (p.77)	Detox Ratatouille (p.93)	Turkey Meatballs with Zucchini Noodles (p.71)
SNACK	Walnut Raisin Banana Bread (p.101)	Cucumber Avocado Rolls (p.120)	Baked BBQ Plantain Chips (p.127)	Walnut Raisin Banana Bread (p.101)	Cucumber Avocado Rolls (p.120)	Walnut Raisin Banana Bread (p.101)	Baked BBQ Plantain Chips (p.127)

WEEK 4

BREAKFAST	Veggie Egg Muffins (p.27)	Good For You Hummus Toast (p.22)	Veggie Egg Muffins (p.27)	Ginger Beet Smoothie (p. 109)	Good For You Hummus Toast (p.22)	Veggie Egg Muffins (p.27)	Ginger Beet Smoothie (p. 109)
LUNCH	Turkey Meatballs with Zucchini Noodles (leftover)	Honey Mustard Drumsticks (leftover)	Savory Salmon and Garden Veggie Stew (leftover)	Ground Turkey Stuffed Bell Peppers (leftover)	Garlic-Lime Mahi Mahi (leftover)	Mushroom Risotto (leftover)	Bison Burger with Sweet Potato Fries (leftover)
DINNER	Honey Mustard Drumsticks (p.76)	Savory Salmon and Garden Veggie Stew (p.52)	Ground Turkey Stuffed Bell Peppers (p.67)	Garlic-Lime Mahi Mahi (p.58)	Mushroom Risotto (p.93)	Bison Burger with Sweet Potato Fries (p.77)	Hearty Barley and Vegetable Soup (p.51)
SNACK	Turmeric Ginger Broccoli Bites (p.124)	Lemon Blueberry Cheesecake Bars (p.104)	Coconut-Crusted Tofu Bites (p.121)	Turmeric Ginger Broccoli Bites (p.124)	Lemon Blueberry Cheesecake Bars (p.104)	Coconut-Crusted Tofu Bites (p.121)	Turmeric Ginger Broccoli Bites (p.124)

Tips for Meal Preparation & Staying on Track

Staying consistent matters more than striving for perfection; occasional slip-ups may happen. What is more important is to embrace the imperfect progress, enjoy the journey, and explore new foods while celebrating each small step towards anti-inflammatory wellness. Here are some easy meal prep tips to incorporate into your life:

- **Plan Your Meals Ahead of Time:** Design a weekly menu featuring breakfast, lunch, dinner, and snacks with plenty of vegetables, lean proteins, whole grains, and healthy fats. Use this to shop smarter by focusing on seasonal produce and aligning your grocery list with anti-inflammatory principles.

- **Prep Bases, Not Entire Meals:** Instead of prepping entire meals, focus on preparing versatile bases like roasted sweet potatoes, sautéed mushrooms, or seasoned lentils that can easily be mixed and matched with different proteins and greens throughout the week.

- **Embrace Batch Cooking:** Cook larger quantities of hummus, soups, stews, and casseroles, then freeze portions for future meals. You can enjoy leftovers for lunches or as easy dinners on busy nights when you don't have the energy to cook.

- **Create Portable Snack Packs:** Prepare snack packs with nuts, carrots, veggie sticks with hummus, fresh fruit with nut butter or roasted pumpkin seeds to fend off cravings and stabilize blood sugar. These mini-meals are perfect for on-the-go energy between meals.

- **Cook Once, Eat Twice:** Turn leftovers into entirely new dishes by using last night's grilled chicken in a salad or wrap. This strategy saves time while ensuring you minimize waste and maximize your meal prep.

- **Sprout Your Legumes:** As a nutritious salad base try soaking and sprouting beans like lentils and chickpeas, this makes them easier to digest, boosts nutrient absorption, and adds easy crunch to salads or bowls. Store in an air-tight container in the fridge.

- **Rotate Your Greens:** Instead of sticking to the same greens, switch between kale, arugula, dandelion greens, and Swiss chard. This provides different phytonutrients and keeps your salads exciting.

- **Create Infused Oils:** Infuse olive oil with garlic, rosemary, or lemon zest to drizzle over grilled vegetables, salads, or roasted fish for a quick hit of flavor.

- **Dehydrate Fruits and Veggies:** Dehydrated apples, zucchini, and tomatoes can be homemade snacks or crunchy salad toppers that add texture without preservatives.

- **Blend Legumes into Smoothies:** Chickpeas and white beans blend well with fruits like bananas and mangoes to create creamy, fiber-rich and filling smoothies.

- **Stay Flexible:** Adjust your weekly menu to fit your cravings and mood, keeping versatile ingredients like eggs, greens, and canned tuna for frittatas or salads. This flexibility ensures you can whip up anti-inflammatory meals even when plans change.

- **Plan for Texture Diversity:** When planning your meals, think about the textures of different foods. Combining creamy avocados with crunchy roasted chickpeas or pairing nutty quinoa with fresh, crisp cucumbers creates an appealing experience that makes healthy meals exciting.

- **Embrace International Flavors:** Draw inspiration from global cuisines. Middle Eastern tahini dressings, Mediterranean lemon-oregano marinades, or Indian turmeric-spiced dals add unique flavors to your meals, making it easier to diversify your palate and stay on track.

- **Batch Cook Spices:** To save time and add depth to your dishes, batch-mix blends like cumin-coriander-turmeric or smoked paprika-garlic powder. Store them in jars for quick access to flavor-packed seasoning.

- **Build a Personalized Pantry:** Stock up on anti-inflammatory pantry staples that align with your unique preferences and sensitivities, such as gluten-free grains, plant-based proteins, or low-sodium broths.

Conclusion

Adopting an anti-inflammatory diet is an exciting adventure towards a better health, increased energy, and deeper connection with your body's unique needs. Throughout this process, you've likely observed how your body responds to different foods, experienced a boost in energy, and noticed a reduction in inflammatory symptoms like joint pain, digestive discomfort, or fatigue. Together in this book, we've delved into the principles of an anti-inflammatory diet, explored the powerful effects of various foods, and created delicious, nutrient-rich recipes that nourish both body and soul.

As you reflect on this transformation, you've embraced nutrient-dense foods that combat inflammation. Choosing whole grains over refined carbohydrates, opting for fatty fish instead of processed meats, and enjoying antioxidant-rich fruits and vegetables have all played a part in your healthier lifestyle. Adding herbs and spices like turmeric, ginger, and cinnamon has not only enhanced your meals but also provided potent anti-inflammatory benefits.

We've celebrated the delight of flavorful meals that are both healing and delicious! The recipes here are more than just dishes—they're tools for building a healthier you. Remember, eating for health isn't about perfection; it's about progress. Sometimes convenience or cravings may lead you off course, but every mindful choice you make contributes to your overall well-being. Flexibility is crucial for sustaining this diet. Life is ever-changing, and your approach should be adaptable.

The conclusion of this book is not an end but the beginning of a lifelong commitment to health. With each thoughtful meal, movement, and moment, you're laying the groundwork for a future filled with vibrancy. So, continue to explore, adapt, and savor this path towards a long-term wellness. Your body will thank you every day!

Bonus: The Health Journal

DATE:

M T W T F S S

WEIGHT:

HOURS OF SLEEP:

WATER INTAKE

BREAKFAST:

LUNCH:

DINNER:

SNACK:

GUT HEALTH:

BLOATING (Y/N)

BOWEL MOVEMENT (TYPE, FREQUENCY, DISCOMFORT)

STOMACH PAIN (Y/N)

ACIDITY/HEARTBURN (Y/N)

NAUSEA (Y/N)

EXERCISE:

ENERGY LEVEL (1-10):

3 THINGS I AM GRATEFUL FOR TODAY:

1.
2.
3.

MOOD, SLEEP & STRESS:

MORNIGN MOOD:

EVENING MOOD:

SLEEP QUALITY (1-10)

STRESS LEVEL (1-10)

NOTES ON STRESS TRIGGERS:

PAIN SCALE (1-10):

MORNING PAIN LEVEL:

EVENING PAIN LEVEL:

AFFECTED AREAS:

NOTES ON RELIEF TECHNIQUES:

REFLECTION & GOALS:

1. WHAT WENT WELL TODAY?

2. WHAT CHALLENGES DID YOU FACE?

3. POSITIVE COPING TECHNIQUES USED

4. ONE THING I WILL IMPROVE TOMORROW

5. GOALS FOR TOMORROW (DIET, EXERCISE, STRESS MANAGEMENT)

Appendix 1: Cooking Measurements & Conversions

Dry Measurements Conversion Chart

Teaspoons	Tablespoons	Cups
3 tsp	1 tbsp	1/16 c
6 tsp	2 tbsp	1/8 c
12 tsp	4 tbsp	1/4 c
24 tsp	8 tbsp	1/2 c
36 tsp	12 tbsp	3/4 c
48 tsp	16 tbsp	1 c

Liquid Measurements Conversion Chart

Fluid Ounces	Cups	Pints	Quarts	Gallons
8 fl. oz	1 c	1/2 pt	1/4 qt	1/16 gal
16 fl. oz	2 c	1 pt	1/2 qt	1/8 gal
32 fl. oz	4 c	2 pt	1 qt	1/4 gal
64 fl. oz	8 c	4 pt	2 qt	1/2 gal
128 fl. oz	16 c	8 pt	4 qt	1 gal

Liquid Measurements (Volume)

Metric	Standard
1 mL	1/5 tsp
5 mL	1 tsp
15 mL	1 tbsp
240 mL	1 c (8 fl. oz)
1 liter	34 fl. oz

Dry Measurements (Weight)

Metric	Standard
1 g	.035 oz
100 g	3.5 oz
500 g	17.7 oz (1.1 lb)
1 kg	35 oz

US to Metric Conversions

Standard	Metric
1/5 tsp	1 ml
1 tsp	5 ml
1 tbsp	15 ml
1 fl. oz	30 ml
1 c	237 ml
1 pt	473 ml
1 qt	.95 l
1 gal	3.8 l
1 oz	28 g
1 lb	454 g

Oven Temperatures Conversion

Celsius	Fahrenheit
120 C	250 F
160 C	320 F
180 C	350 F
205 C	400 F
220 C	425 F

1 CUP

1 cup = 8 fluid ounces

1 cup = 16 tablespoons

1 cup = 48 teaspoons

1 cup = ½ pint

1 cup = ¼ quart

1 cup = 1/16 gallon

1 cup = 240 ml

A Heartfelt Note to End On

Congratulations on taking this important step toward a healthier, more vibrant you! Whether you're just beginning or deepening your anti-inflammatory journey, let this be an adventure filled with excitement, flavor, and discovery. Imagine the mouthwatering, nutritious meals you'll create—each bite nourishing your body, mind, and spirit. This isn't just about food; it's about reclaiming your well-being, one delicious, guilt-free meal at a time.

So go ahead—get creative, savor every bite, and trust that you're making choices that fuel your best life. You've got the tools, the recipes, and the power to thrive!

We'd Love to Hear Your Story!

Thank you for choosing *The Anti-Inflammatory Cookbook for Beginners*. Your experience matters, not only to us but to the many others seeking to transform their health through easy, flavorful meals.

If you found joy in these recipes or felt the meal plans made your life just a little easier, we'd be so grateful if you could share your thoughts with the world! A quick review on Amazon goes a long way in helping others discover the transformative power of this journey. Plus, your feedback fuels our passion to keep creating recipes that make a real difference.

Simply scan the QR code below to leave a review—it's quick, easy, and means the world to us! Thank you for being part of this delicious, healthy adventure. Here's to happy, healthy cooking!

Thank you for your support!

Now, go shine! Your journey has just begun!

Printed in Great Britain
by Amazon

56107392R00079